PRAISE FOR EMOTIONAL
FREEDOM TECHNIQUES

~

From the author of *Rx for RNs*, *Take One Breath*, *In This Moment*, and *33 Nurses*, comes *Emotional Freedom Techniques*, a concise guide to using EFT Tapping to relieve stress and its related impacts on mind, body, and spirit.

"Right from the beginning Terry begins by building a foundation of understanding by offering both the science and research of tapping. She then offers practical experiential exercises that gently takes the reader through the tapping process. This book is truly a great resource for anyone new to tapping as well as the seasoned tapper."

— **Mary Ayers**, PhD, EFT Coach, Author, and Speaker

EMOTIONAL FREEDOM TECHNIQUES

The Art of Managing Stress Through EFT Tapping

TERRY MALUK

DEDICATION

～

*May this book bring you a sense of curiosity, possibility, freedom,
and joy as you discover how easy it is to release old baggage you
didn't even know you had.*

CONTENTS

INTRODUCTION

"Once your negative emotions, beliefs, and experiences have been processed and released, you're free to feel and be positive again." – Nick Ortner

---

These are exciting times for anyone seeking proven methods of self-care. We are becoming more aware of and proficient at using techniques we can learn from a professional and then practice on our own in our daily lives. There are books, workshops, courses, and supporting research covering every self-care topic imaginable, teaching alternative and complementary techniques to our existing modes of healing.

One of the most exciting fields of ongoing study and practice is a combination of old and new, east and west, mind and body. It's called Emotional Freedom Techniques (EFT), or EFT tapping, or just tapping. Imagine self-administered acupressure (similar to acupuncture but without the needles) combined with conventional talk therapy. It's a powerful combination that yields remarkable results, as you'll learn for yourself in this book. With the simple practice of tapping, you can take self-care literally into your own hands.

How did I find EFT? My sister-in-law had given me a link to one of The Tapping Solution's first annual summits. For ten days each year, they provide free online presentations from a variety of experts who offer examples of how to use tapping for physical and emotional issues. I watched for a few days but got a little lost because, at that time, I considered tapping a little too "woo-woo" for me.

My background is in science, and back then, I didn't have an interest in learning about an unconventional technique I didn't believe would actually work. However, when the annual summit came around again the following year, I was experiencing extreme stress at work and suffering from chronic low-back pain and migraines. Maybe it was time to listen and give EFT a try.

I was amazed to discover that this tapping thing worked for me. It quickly relieved my physical issues by helping me find and address the root causes of the pain. EFT tapping became part of my stress-relief toolbox, as well as my go-to for mindset work. Other helpful tools I love include breathwork and mindfulness meditation, which you can learn about in the first two books of my *Art of Managing Stress* series: *Take One Breath* and *In This Moment*.

As I practiced tapping more often, I noticed an overall calmer feeling. Tapping helped me neutralize emotional issues as well. I was able to reduce my chronic stress and calmly handle my stress triggers at work and in other areas of my life. I set comfortable boundaries with confidence. And as a result, my physical issues occurred less and less frequently. It's all connected.

This book is for those new to EFT tapping, as well as for those who want to learn more or expand their practice. You'll read about stress and its impact on the mind and body over the long term—and why relieving stress is a good goal.

You'll be guided through a step-by-step approach on how to tap, including a clear diagram of the tapping points. You'll read about success stories made possible with tapping and some of the most common questions about tapping. You'll learn some general approaches to managing stress with EFT as well as some additional tapping techniques for you to test out. You'll learn how to use scripts as starting points on your way to finding your own specific words, and you'll see how easy it can be to manage common stress-induced pains. Suggestions about how to incorporate tapping into your life will hopefully inspire you to discover where you can easily practice tapping each day.

Finally, you'll read about the abundance of existing and ongoing research around EFT tapping; this chapter is near the end of the book in case you want to get started practicing EFT right away without getting distracted. You can always skip ahead to the "Scientific Evidence" chapter if you prefer to see the proof first before coming back to the "EFT Basic Recipe" chapter. I totally understand both approaches. You'll have access to a selected list of references from the extensive body of research and science that proves EFT tapping is an evidence-based modality.

Tapping works for millions of people. It can work for you, too. What have you got to lose by trying it? Maybe it's time to say goodbye to that pain in your neck.

The information in this book is far from comprehensive. There is so much to know about EFT tapping, so much that it can do, and so many subtle uses of the techniques. I hope you take the time to explore further once you become familiar with the basics.

Smile, take a breath, and let's get started.

Please remember: It's important to contact a professional if things feel too big for you. And never discontinue your current medications without first consulting your doctor.

❧ 1 ❧
IS THIS YOU?

"EFT offers great healing benefits." – Deepak Chopra, MD

H ere's a scenario that might sound familiar. You wake up exhausted. Your mind races immediately to all the things you need to do today. You're in a constant rush to get somewhere and to get everything done. You give up on your to-do list and just try to make it through the newest crisis at work or at home. There's no time to fix a healthy meal, so fast-food takeout or pizza delivery is the easiest choice. And of course, you feel guilty about that, so why not have the cookies, too? Running errands in bad traffic on the way home leaves you overwhelmed and frustrated. The chores at home are building up. And then, the washer breaks. By the time the day is done, you're exhausted, but you decide to check your email. Then you can't fall asleep, or you wake up in the middle of the night, going over all the things that went wrong that day. When the alarm goes off, you wake up exhausted....

Sadly, this situation is all too familiar for a growing number of people. Stress has become an expected part of life. When I speak to groups, I'll ask for a show of hands from those who are feeling stressed. Almost every single person raises their hand, nodding their head in understanding. Sometimes we wear our stress like a badge of honor and compare stories about how much of it we have in our lives. I know I've participated in conversations like that in the past.

So, what exactly is stress? The American Institute of Stress[1] defines it this way: "The original definition of stress by Hans Selye, who coined the term as it is presently used, was, 'the non-specific response of the body to any demand for change.' " Through experimentation, Selye found that short-term stressful situations can result in impacts on the stomach, lymph system, and adrenals. He found that chronic or long-term stress can result in heart and/or kidney disease, stroke, and rheumatoid arthritis. He later defined stress as "the rate of wear and tear on the body." Selye's research attracted much attention, and *stress* became a well-used buzzword to describe many situations.

There can be good stress (eustress), such as winning an award, being offered an exciting new job, getting engaged to be married, or buying a house. But stress is most often identified with things that aren't so good (distress): bills, relationship problems, or the boss from you-know-where.

Some say that a little stress in life is useful to help with performance. Nothing like a call from an upset supervisor to motivate you, right? Others disagree, saying any amount of stress is bad. But either way, when you're stressed, you don't do your best creative thinking. When your body is in a fight, flight, or freeze mode because of perceived threats, you aren't at your best for making good choices quickly. Can you imagine doing a math problem while being chased by a tiger? While a looming deadline at work isn't a tiger, your body perceives that deadline as a threat, taking your creative brain offline because stress hormones impact your thinking.

How many times do you keep retelling a stressful story or relive it in your mind? It's been shown that remembering or retelling a stressful event causes the body to react as though the event were happening again. Stress management has become a necessity for many people to avoid health issues, prolonged illness, and insomnia. Chronic stress, day in and day out, at work and at home, is not a good thing. So you must recognize your warning signs and limit how much stress you're exposed to and your reaction to it.

When you sense a perceived danger of any type, your body begins to produce stress hormones. Three major stress hormones include adrenaline, norepinephrine, and cortisol. Adrenaline and norepinephrine help you focus on the threat, making you more aware of it. Your heart and breathing rates increase, your muscles tense, and you may even start sweating. Blood flow shifts from less critical areas, like digestion and analytical thinking, to your muscles, so you can react physically—run—if you need to. You're on high alert of the perceived threat.

The amygdala, the alarm center of the brain, makes a decision based on previous experience to determine whether a situation is a threat. For example, the last time the boss called an emergency meeting with the team, someone was unexpectedly fired.

But once a situation is perceived as nonthreatening, the all-clear signal is given in the brain. Your body begins to return to a resting state, which can take anywhere from thirty minutes to a few days.

If the situation *is* perceived as dangerous, a cascade of signals to other parts of the brain and body produce more chemical reactions, which ultimately result in the production of the stress hormone cortisol, secreted by the adrenal glands. This response is perfect for helping you out of a dangerous situation quickly and efficiently. It's meant to get you through the crisis, after which you can shake it off (animals literally shake to release it) and get back to a resting state.[2] However, when you live in a state of chronic stress, you stew in stress hormones, never getting a chance to return to a healthy rest and digest state.

The body's reactions to this "stress soup" include:

- elevated cortisol levels that interfere with your learning and memory,
- compromised immune function,
- reduced bone density,
- increased weight,
- higher blood pressure and cholesterol, and
- increased risk for heart disease.

You can also experience blood sugar fluctuations and get sick more often. Aches and pains increase. Elevated levels

4

of cortisol, if left unchecked, increase abdominal fat, which is associated with heart attacks and strokes. Studies show that chronic stress and elevated cortisol also increase the risk of depression, mental illness, and can lower life expectancy. These chemicals and the feelings they create can also be addictive. So, while stress isn't good for you, it can leave you wanting another "hit" because you unknowingly crave it.

Previously, a client had trouble making lasting progress on relieving her stress. As we worked together, we made sure she could feel the results of EFT tapping. She agreed to practice, and she experienced some great results. And then, her practice time would decrease until she stopped entirely. What caused her to give up once she started seeing the results of reduced stress? Her body was rebelling because it was addicted to the rush of stress hormones and the familiar feelings she was used to having. Once this concept registered with her, we practiced tapping to address this subconscious self-sabotage quirk. She became aware of her reactions and choices, and she started practicing her tools again with great and lasting success.

All this is scary stuff, and you don't want to get stressed out about being stressed out. So, what do you do when you see warning signs, or worse yet, miss the warning signs and reach a breaking point? Thankfully, there are many helpful methods to reduce stress. Let's start tapping.

THE EFT BASIC RECIPE

"The cause of all negative emotions is a disruption in the body's energy system." – Gary Craig

---

It's time to learn how to use EFT to make your life better starting today. Tapping is a simple yet profoundly powerful technique that's scientifically proven to reduce stress and anxiety. By learning to focus on exactly what is stressing you, and how it's affecting you, you gain clarity and the ability to laser focus on the issue and release the stress more easily. With that comes relief from many seemingly unrelated issues, including physical pain, migraines, weight gain, sleeplessness, phobias, and more.

Sound too good to be true? As you'll read later, tapping has been proven to work by scientists and those who practice it worldwide. Visit the "Scientific Evidence" chapter any time you start to doubt that tapping is not based on repeated scientific research and study.

Are you worried that this will never work for you? You can tap for that! You have so much to gain by committing to try it.

INTRODUCTION TO EMOTIONAL FREEDOM TECHNIQUES

Emotional Freedom Techniques is a straightforward method that can provide stress relief in minutes. One of the best things about tapping is that it's a self-help tool. You can use EFT tapping to reduce stress whenever you choose, and the more you use it, the easier it becomes to recognize and clear any resistance you might have, creating a more calm, peaceful, and rewarding life. Believe it or not, most of us have some subconscious blocks to ridding ourselves of our problems, and tapping can help us get to the bottom of that.

EFT uses gentle stimulation of points on some of the same energy lines, called meridians, used in acupuncture and acupressure (acupoints), combined with the current psychology technique of talk therapy (cognitive behavioral therapy); East meets West. Tapping and talking is easy to do and can provide quick and lasting benefits.

EFT has an interesting history. In the 1970s, the work of psychiatrist Dr. John Diamond, chiropractor Dr. George Goodheart, and psychologist Dr. Roger Callahan led to a surprising discovery. Their patients experienced relief for a variety of issues, including fears, phobias, and stress, by talking about their problems while stimulating acupoints on specific energy lines. Callahan patented the technique, calling it Thought Field Therapy (TFT). TFT was one of the first methods developed in the field of what is now known as Energy Psychology and is considered an effective evidence-based treatment for self-concept, self-regulation, and trauma and stress-related disorders and symptoms.[1]

Gary Craig, a Stanford-trained engineer, was interested in the field of personal development and studied the work of Dr. Callahan. As Craig realized the potential of this approach, he worked to refine and simplify Callahan's TFT techniques while maintaining positive, measurable results: an evidence-based methodology. He ultimately developed a simple and effective set of techniques he called EFT, which he made available freely on his website in the 1990s.[2]

Since then, EFT has continued to undergo rigorous testing and refinement by many individuals, groups, hospitals, and universities. Publications in highly respected, peer-reviewed journals continue to support Craig's findings and techniques. Craig's "Gold Standard EFT" is considered to be the original or classic version of EFT.

Groups such as EFT International[3] (formerly AAMET International), EFT Universe[4], the National Emotional Freedom Techniques Training Institute (NeftTI)[5], and others have developed EFT training and certification options for those interested in pursuing the use of this tool to help themselves and others.

HOW TAPPING WORKS

As mentioned earlier, when you experience or even recall something stressful, the fight, flight, or freeze alarm goes off in your brain. In an efficient cascade of physiological responses, that alarm causes stress hormones to be produced that help you fight, run, or freeze to avoid danger. Usually, the perceived danger doesn't warrant a full-out alarm response. Often, it's just a memory. But your body reacts as though it's happening in the present moment. The result is that you're frequently exposed to stress hormones unnecessarily. This repeated exposure is not good.

When stress hormones are circulating in your system, they slow or stop digestion, compromise your rational thinking, and reduce the effectiveness of your immune system. When you live in a chronically stressed condition, you can expect to see physical and emotional consequences.

And this is where EFT tapping comes in.

Gentle stimulation via tapping on specific points on your hand, head, and torso sends a calming signal to the alarm center in the brain that all is well, even though the threatening thought is still present. The specific points used in EFT coincide with known acupoints on your body's energy lines. The understanding is that tapping on these points disrupts and removes energy blockages and releases stress from your body's energy system. Gary Craig's EFT Discovery Statement is, "The cause of all negative emotions is a disruption in the body's energy system."[6] With repeated tapping, your brain finally gets the message: this thing that was previously filed as "dangerous" is not a threat. Your energy balance is restored, and you return to a healthier state both physically and emotionally.

HOW TO TAP

The easiest way to learn how to tap is to use Craig's "basic recipe," which includes the specific tapping points on the body and the different statements said while tapping. The basic recipe also includes estimating the intensity of your physical or emotional discomfort before and after tapping, so those levels can be compared to measure your progress. It might sound complicated, but it's very simple.

Once you've practiced EFT tapping even a little, you'll more easily find your own words to indicate what you're feeling, which will be most beneficial to you. It's crucial to use words that describe *precisely* what you're feeling and where you're feeling it in your body to get the quickest and most long-lasting results.

Let's take this step-by-step with an example:

1. First, *focus on an issue* that's bothering you right now. It could be physical or emotional. Be as specific as you can with your description. For this example, we'll be focusing on a specific stressful event: "That stressful argument I had with my supervisor."

2. Next, *estimate the intensity level* of the stress you're feeling about that event or issue on a scale from 0 to 10, where 0 is no stress at all and 10 is maximum stress. I recommend keeping a dedicated tapping notebook or journal where you can record your intensity levels both before and after tapping for comparison to check your progress.

3. Then begin tapping on the *side of the hand* point, located on the fleshy area between the base of the little finger and the top of the wrist, with two, three, or all four fingers of the opposite hand. (See the image of the EFT tapping points.) While gently tapping on the *side of the hand* point, say a *setup statement*, which has two parts. The first part includes an acknowledgement of the problem and the second part includes a statement of self-acceptance. For example: "Even though I feel stressed and upset about that argument I had with my supervisor, I accept myself anyway." *Repeat the setup statement three times* while continuously tapping on the *side of the hand* point.

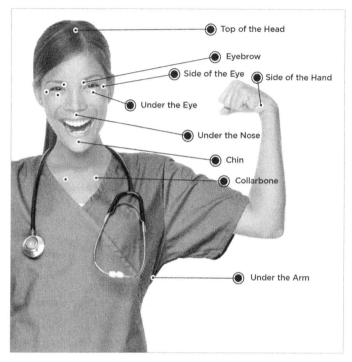

EFT Basic Recipe Tapping Points

4. After the *setup statement*, tap on the *other eight tapping points* shown in the image. With your fingertips or a flat hand, gently tap on each of the other points, one at a time, while saying a *reminder phrase*: a few words or a brief phrase that reminds you of the problem. For example: "That stressful argument with my supervisor." The number of times you tap isn't critical, so don't worry about counting them. Just tap and talk.

- Start tapping gently on the *top of the head* point while saying your *reminder phrase*: "That stressful argument with my supervisor."
- Continue to the next point, which is the *eyebrow* point, on the inner edge of the eyebrow right where the eyebrow starts. You can tap on either or both *eyebrow* points with one or two fingers. Gently tap while saying your *reminder phrase*: "That stressful argument with my supervisor."
- Next, tap gently on the bone at the *side of the eye* point, either or both eyes, while saying your *reminder phrase*: "That stressful argument with my supervisor."
- Then, follow the bone around and tap gently *under the eye* (either or both) while saying your *reminder phrase*: "That stressful argument with my supervisor."
- Now tap just *under the nose* above the top lip while saying your *reminder phrase*: "That stressful argument with my supervisor."
- Next, tap on the *chin* point, which is in the crease under your bottom lip and above your chin, while

saying your *reminder phrase*: "That stressful argument with my supervisor."

- Then, find the v-notch at the base of your *collarbone*. Move down and out about an inch or so to find the slight indentations there. You can tap on either or both sides. I like to gently tap the whole area with an open hand. Tap there while saying your *reminder phrase*: "That stressful argument with my supervisor."
- Finally, tap about four inches *under the arm* on the side body, either or both sides, while saying your *reminder phrase*: "That stressful argument with my supervisor."

You've just completed one round of EFT tapping! I know it seems like a lot to remember when you're first learning, but I promise it quickly becomes second nature after only a few rounds of practice.

5. After tapping on all those points, *take a slow, comfortably deep breath* and *notice your intensity level again* on a scale from 0 to 10. Write it down next to the initial number for comparison.

6. If your intensity level is still above 3, continue tapping more rounds with new or more specific words until your intensity is as close to 0 as possible. Start at the *side of the hand* point with a new *setup statement* such as "Even though I still have some remaining stress about the argument, I accept myself anyway." Then tap at the *top of the head* point and go through all the points again as many times as you like. You can ask yourself what's keeping your intensity above 0, and then you can tap on that!

You don't need to worry about getting this exactly right. With practice, it becomes more natural and you'll know what is right for you.

Once you're familiar and comfortable with the steps of the basic recipe, you might notice you want to tap longer on one spot than the others. That's fine to do. Follow your instincts. You can keep saying the same *reminder phrase* at each point, or you can change it as different thoughts or words come to you; however, keep your focus on what's bothering you for the first few rounds. You won't reinforce the negative thoughts and emotions by saying them aloud. Instead of continuing to ignore them, you're acknowledging them while at the same time signaling your body that you're safe and that it's okay to release them.

As you tap, your mind relaxes. Old memories may come to the surface, or sudden insights on why you're feeling a certain way might appear. Keep your notebook handy to write down thoughts and recollections so you can tap on them later.

PUTTING IT ALL TOGETHER

Let's practice tapping using the basic recipe with a simple example to experience how easy it is. Have you ever felt stressed about an upcoming meeting? Tapping can help with that.

When you think about an upcoming meeting, do you feel the stress in your body? Notice the sensations you are experiencing in your body. How intense is the feeling of stress, from 0 to 10? Write that number down as your starting point.

Start by saying a simple *setup statement* while tapping on the *side of the hand* point:

> "Even though I'm stressed about this meeting, I accept myself and how I feel."

> "Even though I'm stressed about this meeting, and I feel it in my body, I accept myself anyway."

> "Even though I'm stressed out about this meeting, right now I'm okay."

Then tap on the other points with *reminder phrases*:

> *Top of the Head (TOH)*: "All this stress about this meeting."
> *Eyebrow (EB)*: "And I feel this stress in my body."
> *Side of the Eye (SE)*: "Every time I think about it,"
> *Under the Eye (UE)*: "I get stressed out."
> *Under the Nose (UN)*: "And then my body reacts to this stress."
> *Chin (Ch)*: "All this stress."
> *Collarbone (CB)*: "I feel it in my body."
> *Under the Arm (UA)*: "And I don't do well in meetings when I'm stressed."

Take a slow, comfortably deep breath after this one round of tapping and notice your intensity. Did it go down? Write down your new intensity level and continue with more rounds of tapping if it's still above 3. To get better results, use specific words that describe the meeting, where you feel it in your body, the sensations you feel, and anything else that comes up about the situation that increases your stress. You can tap and talk about how you're feeling while moving from point to point, as though you were talking to a friend.

In the following tapping script, fill in the blanks with specific names or situations, and any sensations you notice in your body, etc.

Tapping on the *side of the hand* point:

> "Even though meetings with _____ always stress me out, I accept myself anyway."

> "Even though I'm stressed about this meeting, and I feel that stress in my _____, I accept myself and how I feel."

> "Even though this stress makes me feel _____, I accept myself anyway."

Tapping through the other points:

> *TOH*: "This meeting with _____."
> *EB*: "Why do I even have to go?"
> *SE*: "I feel this stress in my _____."
> *UE*: "And it feels _____."
> *UN*: "I wonder if it's possible"
> *Ch*: "to release some of this stress,"
> *CB*: "so I can be my best self at the meeting."
> *UA*: "I'm ready and willing to release this stress."

Continue tapping and talking until you've gotten it all out. Take another slow, calming breath and estimate the intensity of the stress now. Write the new number in your notebook. Did your intensity change? Did anything else come up?

The simple steps above represent the foundation of EFT tapping using Gary Craig's basic recipe. You can make remarkable progress on many issues using this simple method. Later in the book, you'll learn a few additional tapping techniques for more stubborn issues.

WHY SHOULD I WRITE THINGS DOWN?

It's a good idea to make a note of your intensity before and after each tapping session so you can keep track of how well tapping is working for you. It's also a good idea to write down the issue or emotion, feeling, or sensation you're tapping for. Here's why.

In a private coaching session, one of my clients had a very emotional issue to work through. As we talked briefly about the issue, I took notes of her specific words to use for her *setup statement* and *reminder phrases*. I took care to make notes about how she felt because using her specific words is what gets the best results. I asked what her current level of intensity about that issue was. She exclaimed, "Oh, it's a 10!" She had no doubt about that intensity, so I wrote it down as the starting point.

Because her intensity was a 10, to keep her safe, we started tapping on the general feeling she had before going more in-depth and using her specific words. (I highly recommend doing this general tapping if you are ever tapping for something with an intensity greater than 8. It takes the initial edge off gently and safely.) After three rounds using her specific words, I could see a change in her face and body posture that signaled she was releasing the negative emotion. She even yawned, which is an excellent sign of release you may experience as well. After we finished those three rounds, I checked in with her about her intensity level. Her words were, "It's a 0. It really wasn't bothering me that much to begin with." I showed her my notes where she reported it was a definite 10, and she was surprised; this is a common result when tapping.

I explained to her that as she taps, she's able to relax, and a change in her system occurs, which unblocks the negative energy. Once that energy is released, she's no longer holding on to the stress or intensity of the event and may even think it was never stressful to begin with. I've experienced this myself, so I'm always glad to have the proof of my initial intensity level, which I always write down before I start tapping. So, remember to write down your intensity levels before and after so you can see how much progress you make as you tap!

A QUICK SUMMARY

Can you see the potential for using EFT tapping to manage stress and overwhelming issues? Tapping can be used for everything!

Here is a summary of the **basic recipe** steps:

1. Identify an issue.
2. Write down the initial intensity level from 0 to 10.
3. Say your *setup statement* three times while tapping on the *side of the hand* point.
4. Say your *reminder phrases* while tapping on the other eight points.

5. Estimate your new intensity level and write it next to your initial intensity level.

6. Continue with more rounds of tapping using the same or new words until the intensity is down to 0 or as close as you can get.

I hope you will allow yourself time to practice EFT tapping daily and keep a notebook or journal of your results. Start with five minutes each day and practice for as long and as often as you want. Use the basic recipe for guidance as needed. If you get stuck, tap without words and see what happens! You'll find this new tool pays off in big and sometimes surprising ways.

Now you have an easy tool to help you progress from stressed to calm. Visit the "Scientific Evidence" chapter any time you start to doubt that tapping can work. You can even tap on your doubt!

In later chapters, you'll discover a few simple scripts to use while learning to tap and searching for your own words, and for tapping on specific issues. There are so many ways you can use EFT tapping now that you have the basics.

USING TAPPING SCRIPTS

While the use of tapping scripts is common in the world of EFT, the opinions on the use of scripts are many. Some EFT practitioners discourage the use of scripts because you aren't using your own specific words. The concern is that pre-written scripts may be too generic for the user to realize real and lasting results; this is a valid concern if one only ever used generic scripts.

Other practitioners encourage the use of scripts, so you have a good foundation from which to explore; this is also a valid viewpoint based on my experience with new clients feeling like they didn't know what to say when tapping. Many times they wouldn't even try tapping on their own simply because they didn't know what to say. Once they had some basic scripts to start with, they were comfortable substituting their own specific words and creating their own *setup statements* and *reminder phrases*.

While I'm providing some scripts for you to learn the basics of EFT tapping, I *highly* encourage you to substitute the words in the scripts with your own words as soon as possible. This way, you'll learn to trust yourself more during your tapping practice and experience better results. The scripts are kind of like training wheels—don't become dependent on them. Have faith in yourself to find and use your own words.

✿ 3 ✿
DOES TAPPING REALLY
WORK?

"EFT has been reported successful in thousands of cases covering a huge range of emotional, health and performance issues. It often works where nothing else does." – Brad Yates

---

In this chapter, you'll read a short collection of stories about how EFT tapping works for a variety of issues. These are experiences based on my work coaching clients individually. The results range from *modest changes* to *significant improvements* to *complete turnarounds* of attitude and emotions. Every client ended their session feeling better than when they began.

No personally identifiable information is given in these stories. Names used are fictional and do not represent clients' real names.

- Bonnie came in with a persistent **pain** behind her

23

right shoulder blade. She described the pain as sharp, with an intensity of 6 out of 10. After several rounds of tapping, the pain moved around to her mid-back but was less sharp with an intensity of 4. We tapped the back pain down to a 2. What came up after tapping was the stress she felt after having driven in traffic and nearly been late for an appointment. We tapped about her fear of being late. An initial intensity of 7 surprised her. After several rounds using her words about disappointing others and disappointing herself, the intensity dropped from 7 to 1. Her pain in both her shoulder and her back was gone, and she laughed about how quickly the tapping worked. Being able to release the blocked energy around being a disappointment to herself and others eliminated the physical pain and kept it from coming back.

- Tammy had been introduced to EFT at a workshop I gave. She used EFT very successfully for herself during her preparation for surgery both before admission and while in the hospital. She found tapping to be an effective self-care tool to relieve **fear** and the resulting tightness in her body. Post-surgery, Tammy was experiencing constipation and fear of having a bowel movement because it might hurt. We had a short session on the phone where we tapped for about 20 minutes, focusing on the fear of pain in the area of surgery if she "let go" and had a bowel movement. Her fear intensity dropped from 8 to 2. The next morning, I received an email from Tammy that she was able to have a successful movement, totally without pain, right after our call the night before!

- Dee wanted to control her **food cravings**. As we tapped on "feeling deprived" if she didn't give in to her cravings, things came up about her work situation and lack of support from her boss. It surprised her that emotions around work could cause food cravings. We tapped on feeling unsupported, and the intensity dropped from an 8 to a 2. After our session, she decided on a process to improve communications with her boss. Dee set a goal to prepare for her conversation with her boss by tapping so she could be strong and calm when letting her boss know how she felt and what she needed. Follow-up: the conversation with her boss went well, and she no longer felt deprived if she didn't have her favorite food. Dee was back in control of when and how much she ate. She also felt more confident and empowered at work!

- Laura also presented with a desire to control her **food cravings**. After tapping on her craving for a particular brand of gummi bears (intensity started at a 10), she recalled a forgotten childhood memory of her mother purchasing that brand for a special occasion. She became emotional with relief and experienced a good release of blocked energy as she remembered the good times with her mother (now deceased). Her craving intensity dropped to a 3, and she promised to tap more that evening to continue reducing the intensity. The next week, she reported wanting one, and only one, instead of the whole bag, and she gave herself permission for that one. Two months later, she still had complete control over how much and when she ate gummi bears.

- Mollie was 84 and presented with back **pain**. She was incredibly open-minded and ready to learn more about EFT tapping. We tapped as we talked about when and where she experienced pain; this helped her become familiar with all the points as she followed along with me. We made good progress on the back pain almost immediately. She described the pain (red, sharp, when she walks) and we tapped using those specific words. Her intensity decreased from an 8 to a 1 after about 4 rounds. She was surprised and delighted at the quick results. Follow-up: Mollie continues to use tapping on her own to relieve pain. She also says it makes her feel happier when she taps.

- Nichole had a working knowledge of EFT tapping and came to work on her **stress** about a testing situation at work. Even thinking about the tests caused her intensity to increase to an 8. We tapped about several specific aspects of the testing scenario that triggered her "brain freeze," using her exact description. Eventually, Nichole started to laugh when we tapped, saying, "I HAVE to be stressed." She shifted on a few of the aspects all at once, and her intensity dropped to a 1. During a second session, we addressed more work issues around the fear of being ridiculed by her team regarding mistakes she might make. We tapped about how she might respond to any ridicule. Nichole created calm responses to practice so she could use them if needed. She uses the finger points (see "Additional Tapping Techniques" chapter) at work often now because it's invisible and it really helps her. Her stress around work issues have faded!

- Tom presented with long-term shoulder **pain** and tightness. After introducing the technique, we talked about the history of the pain, gently tapping as we talked. What came up included some family, relationship, and work issues that happened in the six months prior to the pain starting. We focused first on one family issue that was the most intense and then tapped on aspects related to a specific exchange of words with a family member. After about four rounds, Tom smiled as we made progress, and I asked what events he was recalling while tapping. He said that the incident really didn't seem important anymore, and his intensity had decreased from a 9 to a 0. Tom agreed to create a list of other specific incidents that needed addressing and to continue tapping on his own.

- Rosemary presented with low back **pain**. We began with an introduction to EFT and some specific breathing techniques, and then we tapped first on the pain itself. We "chased the pain," which means as we tapped for pain in one location, it moved to another location. (See more

on the Chasing the Pain Technique in the
"Additional Tapping Techniques" chapter.) We
began with her back (initial intensity of 6,
described as constant burning, sometimes
stabbing, the size of a golf ball). The pain moved
to her glutes (initial intensity of 4), then moved
again to her lower abdomen (initial intensity of 4).
All physical pain points were tapped down to 2.
After introducing the 9 Gamut Procedure (see
"Additional Tapping Techniques" chapter), all pain
intensity dropped to 0.

- Colleen and I were at a gathering and started
talking about EFT tapping. She mentioned she
had a **headache** that had been hurting for about
two hours. I offered to show her EFT in a quiet
space, and she agreed. After a quick introduction
to the technique, we tapped on the physical
sensations of her headache for a few rounds, using
her words of "this red, sharp pain in the right side
of my head." Her headache intensity dropped
from 6 to 2. We tapped and talked about some
worries Colleen had about her brother's health,
stopping to tap on any specific aspect of her worry
that triggered her intensity. She was amazed that
it only took four rounds of "this tapping thing" to
completely relieve her headache, as well as
decrease her worries about her brother.

- Leslie wanted to use EFT tapping to help increase
her level of **self-esteem and self-acceptance**.
When asked about the level of intensity of her
feelings of low self-esteem, she replied, "Off the

charts." As we tapped, we said, "I am open to the possibility of accepting myself," as the affirmation in the *setup statement*. The first time she said those words, she became emotional, so we kept tapping and used that phrase as a *reminder phrase*. She was soon able to say, "I am open to accepting myself," and after two rounds of repeating the statement, she successfully said, "I accept parts of myself." We tapped and talked about viewing herself as a successful person, and she replied, "I don't see myself there." After another round of tapping, using that exact phrase, she suddenly said aloud, "Why not?" She needed time to think about what she had just said, so we tapped together through the points for three rounds without words. After a deep sigh, she said she felt stronger and more confident that she could be successful.

These success stories represent only a small number of those I've witnessed. Most clients visit for multiple sessions, which allows specific issues to be targeted and additional techniques introduced.

There are many more success stories available on Gary Craig's website[1] and the EFT Universe website.[2]

EFT tapping does indeed work for a wide variety of issues. May these success stories encourage and inspire you on your tapping journey.

❄ 4 ❄
WHAT IF ...?

"Everything is energy and that's all there is to it. Match the frequency of the reality you want and you cannot help but get that reality. It can be no other way. This is not philosophy. This is physics." – Albert Einstein

---

Now that you've learned the basics of how to practice EFT tapping and have had a chance to try it, you may have some questions. There are several I answer frequently, so let's address them here.

WHAT IF I DON'T WANT TO TAP?

Maybe you're new to tapping and not quite ready to try it. Or perhaps you've experienced some of the benefits from a session or two and find yourself reluctant to use EFT tapping any further. Either way, here's a gentle challenge for you.

Ask yourself, "Why don't I want to tap?" Let yourself sit quietly with this question for a minute or two, and your mind will start to give you some hints. Create a list of the reasons in your tapping journal.

Here is a sample of responses I've heard from others:

1. It won't work for me.
2. I'll look silly.
3. I don't know what to say when I tap.
4. I might do it wrong.
5. There are too many things to tap about and I don't know where to begin.
6. It's a little scary to bring things up that I don't want to think about.
7. What if it works and I end up changing?

These are all excellent reasons, and EFT tapping can help you to get to the core of each one. I recommend you try one round of tapping on the statement, "I don't want to tap." Estimate how strongly you feel about not wanting to tap, on the 0 to 10 scale, and start tapping: (See the "EFT Basic Recipe" chapter for an image of the tapping points.)

"Even though I don't want to tap, I accept myself."

"Even though I don't want to tap, I forgive myself."

"Even though I don't want to tap, I deeply and completely accept and forgive myself."

TOH: "I don't want to tap. "
EB: "Who knows what might happen. "

32

SE: "If anything happens at all."
UE: "I just don't want to tap, okay?"
UN: "I don't want to tap."
Ch: "I don't want to tap."
CB: "I don't want to tap."
UA: "I don't want to tap!" (Emphasize your words this time.)

Now take a slow, calming breath and check in with your intensity again. Chances are you'll feel a little less resistant and may even wonder what the big deal was. But if you still feel strongly, tap more rounds by going back to the *top of the head* point and start talking about why you don't want to tap. As you tap and talk, reasons may come to mind that might not have been obvious before, and then you can tap on those reasons.

For the seven reasons listed above, or any reason that feels true to you, tap on those words or your specific variation. "Even though it won't work for me ...", "Even though I'll look silly ...", "Even though I don't know what to say ...". By tapping and talking about each reason you have, your intensity level around that reason will go down. After tapping on these and similar statements, clients often say, "It doesn't feel like a big deal anymore. I can try tapping and see what happens." By tapping and talking about these reasons, you become better at tapping, and you'll more likely want to continue tapping!

Touching briefly on the seven reasons above:

1. *It won't work for me*. While not every technique works for everyone and some issues are more

stubborn to resolve than others, when given a chance, tapping can work on most issues.

2. *I'll look silly*. Well, yes, tapping might feel and look a little silly. When I first started tapping, I was too self-conscious to tap in public or even in my car. Once I learned how amazing the benefits of tapping were, I quickly got over the "fear of looking silly" (and yes, that was a tapping topic for me, too.) Now, I regularly tap in the car and during my walks. Besides, with millions of people worldwide using tapping as a self-help tool, many people will recognize the activity. And you're setting a good example for them too. More people tapping means less stress in the world, and that's a good thing!

3. *I don't know what to say when I tap*. This statement is true for everyone when first starting out, which is why I provide some scripts to get you started. Once the tapping process becomes second nature to you, the words will come easier. Just say what you're feeling. And if no words come, tap without words.

4. *I might do it wrong*. The truth is EFT tapping is a very forgiving tool. There are many variations of the basic recipe that have been developed by practitioners since Gary Craig first introduced tapping, and the results are still great. Nick Ortner from The Tapping Solution lists five mistakes that people make regarding tapping: not using it enough, using words that aren't specific enough, not tapping on all the aspects of an issue, not tapping long enough, and not keeping a list of things to tap on.[1] But these mistakes don't mean

you're doing it *wrong*. They just might keep you from getting the best results. The only thing that would be considered "wrong" is trying to work through a "Big T" traumatic event on your own. You should always work with a certified EFT practitioner when addressing serious trauma.[2]

5. *There are too many things to tap about and I don't know where to begin.* Start where you are by tapping on that statement itself. That should calm you enough so that you can make a list of the first things you want to address. Then you can prioritize them. Tap on one or two items each day. Just think, even if you had two hundred issues on your list, you could resolve them all in less time than you think. One of the fantastic things about tapping is that when you work on one issue, it will often neutralize the emotions behind other issues on your list. So if you have a daily practice, it won't take long at all. See the Personal Peace Procedure in the "Additional Tapping Techniques" chapter for more information. Start today!

6. *It's a little scary to bring things up that I don't want to think about.* You've probably heard the phrase "sweeping things under the rug." If something keeps accumulating under the rug, it'll always be there, and you'll always know it's there—even if it's in your subconscious mind. You can't heal what you don't reveal. So start gently tapping on what you're feeling and see what comes up. Again, if it's a traumatic event, please consult with a certified EFT practitioner to address it safely.

7. *What if it works and I end up changing?* Tap on the words: "What if it works?" Let yourself consider

the results of releasing old, negative feelings and emotions, old fears, old beliefs, and old programs holding you back. You may be able to release a chronic pain. You may be able to refrain from binging on certain foods. You may end up being a different person with a more positive outlook, someone who sleeps better, is healthier, and experiences more joy each day. This sounds like a good change to me.

WHAT IF I CAN'T SAY I ACCEPT MYSELF?

Remember the *setup statement* you used when starting the basic recipe? It has two parts. As EFT developer Gary Craig describes them, the first part includes your acknowledgment of the specific problem. The second part affirms your acceptance of yourself despite the problem: "I deeply and completely love and accept myself." How does it feel to say that aloud? Does it feel true?

If you have no problem with those words, continue using them as long as they feel comfortable and true for you. You may want to look at some alternative statements below in case you encounter a tapping situation that causes you to feel less comfortable stating love and acceptance of yourself.

You might be so worked up about an issue that it's hard to say those words aloud, or it might be hard to feel they're true. Maybe it's always hard to say them. If so, try something a little different. Consider these options to complete the *setup statement*: "Even though I have all this stress,"

"I'm open to someday accepting myself."

"I'm willing to consider accepting myself."

"I accept how I feel."

"I can someday accept myself without judgment."

"It might be safe to accept myself."

"I choose to try to accept myself."

"I'm willing to accept myself."

"I allow myself to accept myself."

"That's just how it is for me right now."

"I'm doing the best I can."

"I'm okay."

"Even though I have a hard time saying I accept myself, I accept myself anyway."

You have many options to choose from, depending on how you're feeling. Give yourself permission to use your own words that are positive and true for you. The goal is to reach the point where you can say something positive at the end of your *setup statement*. As you keep saying it, perhaps it will eventually sink in as truth in your heart. At least try to be open to that possibility! And breathe. Now is a great time to practice breathing in feelings of calm and self-acceptance.

Everyone has weaknesses and limitations. Some days, you might not be willing to state your self-acceptance aloud. But if you try first using EFT tapping on the general feeling of not accepting yourself, it can help release the panic and distress, calming yourself enough to do more specific tapping work. That's progress!

There is an abundance of helpful videos and websites with EFT tapping scripts available. You may find even stronger positive acceptance statements, including, "I deeply and completely love, accept, and forgive myself." If you can say that, excellent! If not, substitute it with a positive affirmation truer for you.

WHAT IF I GET STUCK AND DON'T KNOW WHAT TO SAY?

Don't panic. Just keep tapping on the points without words. Or keep tapping, and at each point say things such as:

> "I don't know what to say."
> "I have no words."
> "I can't think of any words."
> "I don't know the right words."
> "I don't know what else to say about this."
> "I just don't know what to say."

Eventually, you'll feel a release of the original emotion or sensation, and the words will come to you.

If the lack of words is frustrating, tap on that:

> "Even though I feel frustrated and don't know what to say, I accept myself anyway."

Use any words that describe the feelings you're experiencing. Those will be the right words.

WHAT IF I DON'T WANT TO SAY ANYTHING NEGATIVE?

Many people are uncomfortable talking about negative feelings and issues because they worry it will reinforce the negative or tap it into their subconscious. The truth is that the negative feelings already exist in the subconscious, and they will remain there until neutralized, no matter how many positive statements are made.

EFT tapping is an excellent way to unblock and neutralize negative feelings. Tapping while talking about them sends a signal to the brain that all is well even though we have these negative feelings, and that it's safe to let them go. If we ignore the problem and only make positive statements, the clever subconscious will secretly undermine our positive words with the nagging little doubts that already exist. (See the "Yes, But ..." chapter.)

So, try using the basic recipe, which includes both the negative and the positive in the *setup statement*, and stick with the negative *reminder phrases* until you feel a shift. Once your intensity has dropped below 3, you might try alternating negative and positive *reminder phrases* and see how that feels. There is nothing wrong with using positive phrases while tapping once you have sufficiently addressed and reduced the negative emotions and sensations.

WHAT IF MY FRIENDS AND FAMILY ASK ABOUT IT?

Your explanation of EFT can be as simple or as detailed as you'd like. The most straightforward answer that seems to be universally understood is this: tapping is a relaxation and stress-management technique. Everyone understands the need to relax and manage stress! If they ask how it works, you can say, "It's like acupuncture without the needles." As you become more comfortable and read further about tapping, you can choose to be more detailed with your description. Or you can refer them to the EFT International website as an excellent source of information.

WHAT IF TAPPING DOESN'T WORK FOR ME?

Sometimes tapping doesn't help right away. Try these suggestions to move the needle:

- First, check your words. Are they specific enough? Are they clear descriptions of the emotions you're feeling? Do they accurately describe the places and sensations you're feeling in your body? You can try exaggerating your words to really get the point across to your subconscious. Being precise with your words can make a big difference in your results.
- Try tapping on an issue that has a lower intensity to see how you respond. If you try tackling a major issue on your own right out of the gate, you may have trouble reducing your intensity. You will do much better by starting on something easier first.
- Drink water. Staying hydrated while tapping is essential. As my friend Denise says, "It's thirsty work!" Seriously though, when you tap, keep some water nearby to sip between rounds of tapping. It can make a big difference in moving stuck energy.
- Please don't give up. Try again later or tomorrow. If you give tapping a chance, it can have an enormous positive impact on your life.

WHAT IF I WANT TO TAP ON SOME POINTS MORE THAN OTHERS?

Many people wonder if it's required to tap on ALL the points, and the short answer is "No." When you're first learning EFT, it's best to follow the basic recipe for at least two or three sessions before altering it to focus more on one or two tapping points. But once you've tapped on all the points, saying the *setup statement* at the *side of the hand* point and your *reminder phrases*, using your specific words about the issue on the other eight points, feel free to alter the order or number of points on which you tap.

As you become familiar and comfortable with the EFT basic recipe and start trusting your tapping intuition, you may be drawn to tap longer or more often on one or two specific tapping points. Without going into detail here, each of the points can help release specific emotions. You may intuitively know which points you need to use for the issue you're facing.

For example, when Roger Callahan was developing what became Thought Field Therapy, he was inspired by Chinese medical practices, including healing based on the body's energy system. He studied the various energy lines, or meridians, and how stimulating endpoints on specific meridians could release blockages associated with negative emotions.

There's a famous story about one of his clients, Mary, who had a long-standing and stubborn issue: fear of water. No amount of standard talk or desensitization therapy seemed to help. Her physical symptoms included feeling sick in her stomach when she thought about getting near water.

Knowing the stomach meridian endpoint under the eye was also associated with fear and worry, Callahan experimented by tapping the point under the eye while Mary talked about her sensation. Mary was immediately able to go near and ultimately into the water!

Based on this realization, Callahan developed specific tapping instructions for various issues based on the emotions and sensations presented. TFT is more complicated than what we know of as EFT today. Gary Craig knew he could bring the miracles of this technique to more people by distilling it down. After careful research and experimentation, he created a shortened tapping sequence that could be used for all issues. Eventually, he was able to condense it down further, creating his basic recipe, which includes the *side of the hand* point and the eight points on the head and upper torso shown in the "EFT Basic Recipe" chapter.

If one or two points feel especially soothing when using the basic recipe to tap, it's fine to focus on those points. Sometimes, there are situations when touching the face is not advised for health reasons. In that case, be sure to thoroughly wash your hands before tapping. You can still tap on all the other points and even add in a few extras if you like, such as tapping the wrists together, or holding or tapping the gamut point (described in the "Additional Tapping Techniques" chapter).

WHAT IF THE SENSATIONS I FEEL IN MY BODY MOVE AROUND?

As part of the basic recipe, we take notice of *where* in our body we feel our emotions when we think about an issue.

Many people have common locations in which they feel their issues, such as the stomach, chest, or throat, or it might be the shoulder or neck. As you tap about an issue and describe the specific sensations you're feeling, you may notice the sensation has changed or shifted to a different part of your body; this is a common result of tapping as blocked energy releases. When the pain or sensation moves and you then change the focus of your tapping, it's referred to as Chasing the Pain. As Gary Craig puts it, "We call the process 'Chasing the Pain' because, as we reduce or eliminate one pain (or discomfort), others show up and require EFT for their resolution."[3] Chasing the Pain is one of the Gentle Techniques (see the "Additional Tapping Techniques" chapter) used in EFT.

You can estimate the intensity of the new sensation or new location and begin with a new *setup statement* and new *reminder phrases* that accurately describe what you're feeling and where you feel it. Tap while focusing on and describing the new location or sensation until you feel a shift or release. Then estimate your intensity level after tapping, taking notice of any other changes or insights into the original issue that may have arisen, which provides you with your next topic for tapping.

WHAT IF I DON'T WANT TO SAY IT ALOUD?

There may be times when you don't want to talk about events that have happened, but they still hold an emotional charge for you, and you want to be free from them. Maybe the experience is too personal to talk about with anyone else. How do you get beyond these emotions to neutralize them? How do you let go of the negative impact the event has had on your life?

EFT founder, Gary Craig, developed several methods for gently dealing with such events. One method allows you to remain silent while neutralizing the negative imbalance in the body's energy system. It's called the Movie Technique. You can use the Movie Technique on yourself, but if things are really intense, working with a trained, experienced practitioner can help.

See the chapter on "Additional Tapping Techniques" for a description of the Movie Technique.

❈ 5 ❈
MANAGING STRESS WITH EFT TAPPING

"Tapping is one of the most directed and powerful ways to peel those layers away of chronic stress." – Dr. Mark Hyman

---

M anaging stress is critical for optimizing physical, mental, emotional, and spiritual health, and EFT tapping is one of the best ways to gently reach the root of your stress, so you can let it go. Tapping is a quick way to bring your overall stress level down so that you can enjoy more clarity of thought and action. EFT also provides an effective way of going deeper, peeling away one layer at a time until you neutralize the negative blocks and restore a healthy flow of energy.

Years ago, it was news to me that physical pain and illness could be caused by chronic stress. Like many, my job at the time involved high levels of stress, dealing with staff and budget cuts that were made even worse by increasing demands from management. Frequent headaches became chronic migraines, and my low back pain began limiting my activity. It took chest pains (and my sweet doctor, bless her) to wake me up to the fact that I needed to do something about my stress if I wanted to live a full life.

I started creating a toolbox of stress-management techniques that I could use to regain control of my life. These tools include breathing methods, yoga, meditation, regular exercise, time in nature, living with gratitude, and EFT tapping. I continue to research and read everything I can find about creating a more joyful life, releasing old beliefs that hold me back, and replacing them with new empowering beliefs.

You can use tapping to address many kinds of stress, including work stress, family stress, relationship stress, financial stress, physical health stress, and major life-event stress. I promise once you start using EFT tapping regularly, you'll find that the quality of your life will improve on many fronts, because it's all connected.

I recommend using your tapping journal to start a list of any areas in your life you'd like to start releasing stress. (See the Personal Peace Procedure section in the "Additional Tapping Techniques" chapter.) You can update your list anytime you make progress or encounter new issues. Life is always bringing change. Tapping can help gracefully maneuver whatever comes your way.

After you've made your list, prioritize the items so you know where you'd like to start. Once you've identified your top priority, break it down based on specific events, people, or situations. For example, if it's financial stress, identify what worries you the most. Is it a specific bill? Is there an emotion or feeling that comes to mind? Does it involve a specific person? Does it remind you of anything in the past? Sometimes our stressful situations are invisibly connected, so by identifying the specific pain points of a single issue, you may be able to release multiple issues on your list. EFT is magic like that, helping you creating a safe space to release and let go.

Starting with the first thing you'd like to feel better about, ask yourself some questions. When you think about the situation, what bothers you the most? There may be several things but start with one. Do you feel an emotion or sensation anywhere in your body? How intense is the emotion or sensation? Notice if the emotion or sensation has a color, size, texture, aroma, or makes a sound. Write down your intensity level in your journal.

Begin tapping, using the generic script below, and fill in the blanks with your own specific words to describe the situation and the feelings or sensations. Refer to the basic recipe tapping points image in the "EFT Basic Recipe" chapter as needed.

Start with your *setup statement*:

> "Even though I feel all this stress about _____, and it makes me feel _____, and I feel it in my body in my _____, I accept myself anyway."

> "Even though I am stressed about _____, and I feel it in my _____, I accept myself and how I feel."

"Even though I feel this stress about _____ in my_____, and it makes me feel _____, right now I'm okay."

Then continue with *reminder phrases*:

TOH: "All this stress."
EB: "All this stress about _____."
SE: "I feel it in my _____."
UE: "All this stress!"
UN: "I'm so tired of feeling _____."
Ch: "I feel this in my _____."
CB: "All this stress about _____."
UA: "All this stress."

After this one round of tapping, check in with yourself to see how intense your feelings are. Did anything change? Do you still feel the sensation in the same place in your body? What came up? Did anything else come to mind, such as a memory or new thought about the situation?

If your intensity is still above 3, continue tapping with any additional words or memories that come to mind about the situation. By tapping on the meridian endpoints, you let your brain and body know you're safe. Once the emergency alarms begin to quiet, you may see the next layer of the puzzle. Did the sensation move from one place in your body to another? As mentioned earlier, this is normal. Chasing the Pain allows you to tap specifically for each sensation and location until it is all neutralized. Did the emotion you were feeling change? Again, whether it does or doesn't, this is normal. Simply update your words if needed to match what you're feeling and continue tapping until your intensity is as close to 0 as possible.

Remember the basic recipe steps:

1. Identify an issue.
2. Write down the initial intensity level 0 to 10.
3. Repeat your *setup statement* three times while tapping on the *side of the hand* point.
4. Say your *reminder phrases* while tapping on the other eight points.
5. Guess your new intensity level and write it next to your initial intensity level.
6. Continue with more rounds of tapping, using the same or new words until the intensity is down to 0 or as close as possible.

Sometimes you might get so wound up that you don't even know how to start, or don't want to tap and have to think about what to say. That's okay! Remember, you can just tap on the points without words until you feel a bit better or until the words come. You may want to tap and rant about the situation or the person or how you feel. That's fine, too! Tapping and ranting aloud is another excellent technique for blowing off steam in a safe, calming way. Tapping on the points lets the body know this isn't really an emergency, so it's safe to release the stress and calm down. And with greater clarity that comes from being calmer, you may even discover the truth behind, and a solution to, the problem.

As you become calmer, you may notice hidden emotions and old memories rise to the surface. These sometimes-surprising reminders are helpful clues to what's behind some of your current behaviors and energy imbalances. You may even smile as the lightbulb appears over your head: "Ahhhhh, THAT'S why I do that." As the puzzle pieces start to fall into place around a particular issue, you'll slowly neutralize the blocked energy around it. You might sigh, yawn, or even laugh as the origin of your stress becomes completely obvious. "Why didn't I see that before?" Simply put, it's because you weren't calm enough to see it. You were still in a fight, flight, or freeze emotional state, and there was little, if any, clarity.

While tapping helps you finally see and appreciate the importance of those memories or hidden emotions, sometimes when those memories come up, they're scary and maybe bigger than you're ready to deal with at the moment. If you're tapping on your own, this can lead to discomfort and even panic about what to do with this new information. If you're tapping alone, you can Sneak Away from the intensity of the surfacing emotions. (There's more on Sneaking Away in the "Additional Tapping Techniques" chapter.) Keep tapping on the *side of the hand* point while you repeat the *setup statements*:

> "Even though this is more than I want to deal with right now, I completely accept myself and how I feel."

> "Even though I don't think I'm ready to handle this now, I love, accept, and forgive myself." (Check to make sure that feels true and change the words as needed.)

"Even though I know I need to work on this again later, I love, honor, and accept myself."

Once you've reduced the intensity so that you feel safe and more comfortable, you may want to think about contacting a certified EFT practitioner[1] to help you through these memories and emotions. You don't have to do it alone. Working with a professional can help you restore balance and provide some specific tools to support you through a tough issue.

In the next chapter, you'll learn additional tapping techniques that can help you stay safe and get unstuck as you expand and customize your tapping. And then you'll be given some easy scripts to obtain relief from some of the physical manifestations resulting from chronic stress, such as headaches and back pain.

❧ 6 ❧
ADDITIONAL TAPPING
TECHNIQUES

"EFT is easy, effective, and produces amazing results. I think it should be taught in elementary school." -- Donna Eden

---

Gary Craig named his methods Emotional Freedom Techniques, plural, because he developed multiple ways to address issues. New tapping techniques continue to be added by practitioners worldwide. Humans are wonderfully unique individuals, and what works for each may be a little different. This chapter provides you with a variety of additional tapping techniques that can be used along with the EFT basic recipe.

Some techniques are especially useful in situations where you're not comfortable tapping on your head and body. Some will work when you're stuck at a certain intensity level and want to break through. Some help you approach an issue slowly and safely retreat—if needed. Try out the techniques and see what possibilities await you.

TAPPING ON THE FINGER POINTS

Additional tapping points that aren't usually included in the EFT basic recipe include points on the thumb and each finger. These points can be added to your tapping routine when you encounter stubborn issues, or when you want an easy way to tap anywhere or anytime, even if you're not tapping on all the other points. Finger tapping can also be used on its own as an effective method of creating a daily habit of tapping, bringing you calming benefits each day.

In addition to including it in your regular EFT basic recipe, finger point tapping is convenient if you feel uncomfortable being seen tapping on all the points, such as in a meeting or while running errands or going for a walk or run. Finger tapping is also useful if you're having trouble falling asleep, or having trouble getting back to sleep. Rather than moving around too much by tapping on all the basic recipe points, gentle tapping on the fingers yields good results. With practice, you can even learn to tap on the finger points with the thumb or other fingers of the same hand, minimizing movement.

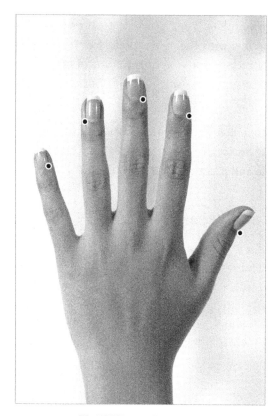

The EFT Tapping Finger Points

The finger points are in the same location on the thumb and three of the fingers, as shown in the image, and on the opposite side of the ring finger. The points are located on the side of the base of the nail. You may see other diagrams of the finger points that either skip the ring finger entirely or show the ring finger point on the same side as the other fingers; this may be done because consistency makes it easier to remember and practice. You can tap either side or even leave out the ring finger, and you will still experience results. But in actuality, the energy line, or meridian, runs down the other side of the ring finger, in line with the gamut point (see below). Therefore, I usually include the ring finger point in my tapping, and I tap on the opposite side or even both sides of the ring finger.

Remember that EFT tapping is a very forgiving technique, so don't worry about getting it exactly right. Follow your intuition and practice what works best for you.

HOLD AND BREATHE

Another way to stimulate the meridian endpoints on the thumb and fingers is to gently squeeze both sides of the base of each nail. Starting with the thumb on one hand, use the thumb and index finger of the other hand to gently hold and squeeze one finger at a time while taking a calming breath. Inhale, exhale, and move to the next finger and gently squeeze both sides. Continue through all the fingers.

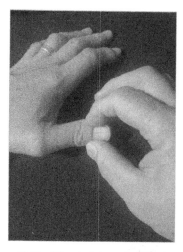

Hold and Breathe Point on the Thumb

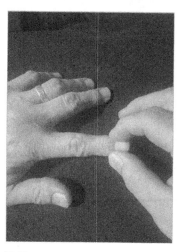

Hold and Breathe Point on the Index Finger

You can then either start again at the thumb of the same hand or change hands and work through the thumb and all the fingers on the other hand, continuing until you feel more at ease. Again, experiment and notice what feels right for you in different situations. Make these techniques your own.

This gentle method of holding the finger points while breathing is also beneficial for improving sleep quality and quantity, and it requires even less movement than tapping on the finger points as mentioned earlier. You can also use this technique anytime to take the edge off as soon as you feel stress building, and it's much less obvious in public situations than tapping. You can be holding one hand with the other while you inconspicuously hold the base of each nail.

I've taught this quick and easy method to several people on flights who are experiencing fear before takeoff. They don't care how or why it works; they just want to feel better. This technique works quickly to control their escalating level of fear, and they always look surprised at how well it works. Once they're feeling more relaxed, that's when the questions start, and I get to talk about the many benefits of EFT tapping.

Clients ask if it's necessary to say the *setup statements* or *reminder phrases* while tapping or holding the finger points. It certainly doesn't hurt if you choose to talk as you practice these techniques. But words are not necessary to experience the benefits of neutralizing negative energy and allowing any blockages to dissolve, so you're back to your best self quickly. If you like, you can say the words to yourself in your mind. Find what works for you and practice often.

BREATHE AND TAP

By taking intentionally slow, comfortably deep breaths, you can reduce stress and its negative impacts on your body. When you're stressed, the resultant quick, shallow breaths rob your body of the benefits that a full breath provides. By adding tapping to your breathing, you increase the power of both tools to yield excellent results. (You can read more about breathing for stress management in the first book in this series, called *Take One Breath*.)

To start, notice your breathing right now while reading this. Are you breathing rapidly or slowly? Are your breaths shallow, or are you breathing deeply? Where do you feel your breath in your body? Where do you feel the expansion in your body?

Take a slow, comfortably deep breath in through your nose. Pause for just a moment with a full breath, and then exhale slowly through your mouth, emptying the lungs. Control your exhale so that it lasts longer than your inhale. As you exhale, release and let go, noticing where you feel tension, relaxing all the muscles in your body. Take two more breaths like that to establish a rhythm.

Now add EFT tapping to your breathing. The easiest way is to start tapping on the *side of the hand* point as you inhale. No words are needed. Tap on the *top of the head* for your exhale, tap on the *eyebrow* point for your inhale, tap the *side of the eye* for your exhale—and continually move through all the points for each inhale and exhale. If you prefer, you can tap on one point for a full breath as you inhale and exhale, then move to the next point. You may even want to tap on the finger points for this process.

To allow the relaxation response to truly settle in, make sure to take at least ten breaths. Breathe steady, keeping the breaths slow and smooth enough to keep yourself from getting dizzy.

Breathe, tap, and notice how you feel. Write down any thoughts, words, memories, or emotions that arise as a result of breathing and tapping, and you can tap on those using the basic recipe when you feel ready.

A variation of this technique is called Touch and Breathe (TAB)[1], where instead of tapping on each point, you simply touch the basic recipe points, take a breath, and then move on to the next point.

SNEAKING UP ON THE PROBLEM

What if you have an emotional issue that feels really big, maybe too big to even say the words aloud, even to yourself? There are several Gentle Techniques for EFT, provided by founder Gary Craig, that are great to help in this situation. One of them is called Sneaking Up on the Problem. You can do this by starting out with very general or even vague thoughts or words about the issue, using similarly vague *setup statements* and *reminder phrases*.

Another Gentle Technique that's helpful when carefully approaching an issue is called Tearless Trauma, which involves "guessing" what your intensity level would be if you simply imagine the issue or if you think about having to describe it. One variation of the Tearless Trauma Technique is to imagine putting the issue into a locked box or treasure chest for safekeeping. You could imagine putting the container behind a curtain or comfortably far away until you're ready to work on the issue. The Box or Container Technique allows you to distance yourself from the problem and gives you a feeling of having some control over the issue and its intensity. (The Box Technique can be used to Sneak Away from the Problem as well, as mentioned in a later section.)

Typically, using very specific words and descriptions when tapping for a problem will yield the best results to help bring an emotion to resolution. But in the case of a trauma, you don't want to be traumatized all over again, so it's best to approach the problem in a more general way to neutralize the immediate feelings of distress. If you're already incredibly stressed, start with several rounds of tapping using very general statements, or even without words, to help calm you.

Once you feel more relaxed from the initial tapping, you may be able to address specific aspects of the trauma one tiny piece at a time, neutralizing each emotional charge while keeping your overall level of distress low.

What do we say when we're using the Sneaking Up on the Problem Technique? Here are some general *setup statements* that can be used to gently address the problem:

> "Even though I can't think about this right now, I accept how I feel and I'm okay."

> "Even though this is too big for me, I completely accept myself anyway."

"Even though I can't tell anyone about this, I accept and forgive myself."

"Even though this terrible thing happened, I completely accept myself."

"Even though I have no idea what to say right now, I accept how I feel and I'm okay."

Try one or all these statements, or you can make up your own general statements that describe how you feel as long as they're gentle enough for you. If the positive affirmation at the end of the *setup statement* is difficult for you to say, try saying it anyway to see how it feels. If it's still difficult to say, try an alternative affirmation, such as:

"I might be open to accepting myself."

"I may choose to love and accept myself one day."

"It's just the way it is for me right now and I accept that."

Once your intensity level decreases, you might feel more comfortable with a more positive affirmation.

Some gentle general *reminder phrases* could follow the key words in your *setup statements*, such as:

"It's too big."

"I can't even think about it now."

"I can't talk about it yet."

"This terrible thing."

"I feel too overwhelmed right now."

Once your overall intensity level lessens, gradually introduce more specific wording about the traumatic event into your tapping. For example,

"Even though there was this car accident in the past, right now, I'm safe."

Tap for several rounds using new wording that is gentle and appropriate for your problem until you feel your intensity level decreasing. If you're feeling calm enough, try tapping on one specific aspect of the event, such as one sight, sound, color, or smell that you remember. Take it slowly and tap on one small thing at a time.

Only proceed if you're remaining calm as you go through each aspect. Honor yourself and know it's okay to stop, breathe, Sneak Away (see below), and try more later. And please remember it's always okay to ask for help.

SNEAKING AWAY FROM THE PROBLEM

What do we do if we reach the end of our tapping session, but we haven't reached the end of our problem? Yikes! Or maybe as we're tapping alone, guiding ourselves through a particular problem, the issue becomes bigger than we expected. Or maybe we're working with a professional, and our appointment time has come to an end before we've fully resolved the issue. There's a tapping technique for that!

Some events take longer than expected to fully explore, identify, and neutralize the negative energy around them. Sometimes unexpected details and intense emotions can come up. And leaving an issue unsettled can be upsetting. Thankfully, there's a way to gently step back from an issue at the end of a session—acknowledging that further work will be done. It's called Sneaking Away from the Problem.

Near the end of your session, you can use the Box Technique (described in the Sneaking-Up section above). Visualize putting the remaining issues into a box or container placed far enough away so that you feel safe, yet close enough to reach when you're ready to work on the them again.

To gently and safely end the tapping session, once you have the concerns tucked securely in a box, tap on the *side of the hand* point. Repeat *setup statements* that express awareness of the unresolved issues that you plan to work on again at a later time. Here are some examples:

> "Even though I know I haven't dealt with all of this, at this moment, I completely love and accept myself anyway."

> "Even though I'm not all the way through this issue yet, I am proud of myself for working on this, and I love and accept myself."

> "Even though I have to come back to work on this again, I accept, love, and forgive myself."

"Even though sometimes I think I'll never get over this, I deeply and completely love and accept myself anyway."

Again, check in with yourself to make sure the positive part of the statement is true for you. You can change them to words that are still positive, yet true for you in the moment.

Additional example *setup statements* from EFT Universe[2] include:

"Even though I still feel terrible, there will be time to work on this later."

"Even though I didn't solve all of this problem today, there's time in the future."

"Even though I've just started to get in touch with this issue, I'll be fine."

"I can put this away and pick it up next time."

If it helps, you can tap through some or all the other tapping points with gentle *reminder phrases*. When you feel finished tapping, look around the room and take several slow, comfortably deep breaths. That's all there is to it. You've gently eased away from the problem and set the intention to return and continue your work later.

CHASING THE PAIN

Another EFT Gentle Technique is called Chasing the Pain. It focuses on following the change of physical sensations and pain rather than directly confronting any emotional issues behind them; this avoids triggering intense emotions while still addressing them gently. As I mentioned earlier, there are many physical manifestations of emotions and chronic stress. You can address yours one by one and make remarkable progress on previously stubborn issues.

It is normal for a pain or sensation to change locations during or after tapping. New pains may arise as the intensity of the old ones are tapped down. Take notice of any specifics about the new sensation or pain, such as size, color, texture, sound, etc. Write down your new intensity level and begin tapping. In this way, you can address the moving pain until the intensity of all locations and sensations have been decreased. Checking in with yourself, you may find the intensity of old emotional baggage reducing without having to address those emotions directly.

Gary Craig explains the technique called Chasing The Pain on his website, including links to a couple of demonstration videos. Notice the attention placed on very specific descriptions of the sensations.[3]

THE MOVIE TECHNIQUE

The Movie Technique allows you to slowly and silently work through a traumatic event as though you were watching a movie on a screen. This technique works well for a particular event that happened, which has specific characters, and a plot with specific words, actions, and aspects, such as smells or tastes, sounds or sights. By breaking an event down into short, specific scenes that last no more than three minutes, you can safely and more easily neutralize the event by taking it one emotional peak at a time. Then you can move on to additional short scenes in the movie if more exist.

Remember that at **any** point if you feel the intensity is bigger than you're ready to handle on your own, please contact an experienced professional to support you. You can still benefit without actually discussing the specific event. By using the Movie Technique, you can keep all the details to yourself, keeping the entire event private if you choose.

Before starting to work through your movie of this event, before even thinking about the event and its details, give the movie a descriptive title that feels safe. For example, an embarrassing event as a child in school might have a title like "My Presentation" or "They Laughed." If just thinking about the title increases your emotional intensity, guess at the level of your intensity from 0 to 10, and begin tapping on the side of either hand, using a *setup statement* like:

> "Even though just thinking about the title of this movie upsets me, I accept how I feel and I'm okay."

Using the basic recipe, tap on the other points with a *reminder phrase*, such as:

> "This 'They Laughed' movie."

See if you can identify any general emotions you're feeling and use those words. For example: "this anger" or "this sadness." Tap through all the points, take a slow, calming breath, and guess your intensity level again. If your intensity is still higher than 3 just thinking about the movie and its title, repeat the tapping sequence. Ideally, you would get to an intensity level of 0 before moving on to silently running the movie in your head.

Then, starting at a neutral place in the movie before the first intense moment of the event, very slowly run the movie in your head, as though you were watching it on a screen from a comfortable distance. At any point you notice your intensity increasing, stop and tap on the reason. Tune in to what you're feeling and where you feel it in your body, rate the intensity, and use words that describe what you're feeling. For example:

"Even though I'm feeling really sad in my heart because they laughed at me, I completely accept myself anyway."

Tap through the other points, using an appropriate *reminder phrase* such as:

"I'm feeling sad in my heart."

Once your intensity about that scene in the movie is below 3, start at the beginning again, before anything intense happens. Slowly run the movie, stopping to tap down every single intense moment. If there are additional events in your movie, carefully move on to the next one, making sure to stop to tap with each increase in intensity. It's important to move slowly enough that you completely neutralize the negative emotions from each emotional peak in this event.

Once you can rewind the movie and play it through in your head without any increase in intensity, you've likely unblocked the negative emotional energy associated with this event. Testing is critical at this point. You can test this out by rerunning the entire movie in your head and exaggerating the sights, sounds, smells, tastes, or any aspects that had been especially intense for you. If your intensity starts rising again, stop and tap on that part of the movie until your intensity is as close to 0 as possible.

Another way to test your results is to "Tell the Story" aloud about the event if you choose. You can say it aloud to yourself or to a professional working with you. If at any point in the story your intensity increases again, stop there and continue using the basic recipe, tapping on what you're feeling, using words that feel right to you, until your story no longer has any charge to it.

THE 9 GAMUT PROCEDURE

While first studying EFT, I read about a process called the 9 Gamut Procedure that Gary Craig included in his original (longer) basic recipe. It involves tapping on a specific point on the back of the hand while concentrating on an issue and going through nine "interesting" steps. The 9 Gamut Procedure works when a person gets stuck or has trouble decreasing the intensity of an issue while using the standard EFT basic recipe.

TERRY MALUK

After learning this technique, I had concerns about my
clients being open to this unusual series of actions. But
after seeing the amazing results from using the process
myself and with others, I decided to add it in whenever
needed, and nobody has complained! The nine steps
include eye movements and other activities that engage
both hemispheres of the brain. Research shows specific
eye movements to be extremely effective in processing
past traumatic memories.

The gamut point is located on the back of either hand,
about an inch or so down from the lowest knuckles,
between the little finger and the ring finger. Find the
hollow space with one or two fingers of the opposite hand,
moving slowly from the knuckles toward the wrist until
you feel a slight indentation. (This spot corresponds to the
Acupuncture meridian called the Triple Heater, or the
Triple Warmer.)

Once you find the point, focus on the issue, and continue
tapping, holding, or rubbing while doing the following
nine steps:

1. Close your eyes.
2. Open your eyes.
3. Keeping your head still, look hard down to the
   right (only your eyes are moving).
4. Still keeping your head motionless, look hard
   down to the left.
5. Slowly roll your eyes in a full circle in a clockwise
   direction, as if you were looking at each hour on
   the face of a big clock. Go slowly enough so you
   notice each hour.

6. Then slowly roll your eyes in a full circle in the opposite direction, seeing each hour on the clock.
7. Hum about five seconds of any song that comes to mind.
8. Count from one to five aloud.
9. Then hum about five seconds again.

Done! This procedure becomes easier once you've done it a few times, so I recommend practicing. The 9 Gamut Procedure can be used on its own anytime you want, or you can add it to the basic recipe. After the *setup statement* and tapping on all the other points, finish up with the 9 Gamut Procedure. Then take a couple of calming breaths and estimate your intensity level. The small amount of extra time and effort it takes to try this procedure is well worth it.

FLOOR TO CEILING EYE ROLL

When you've tapped your intensity level down to 1 or 2, try adding the Floor to Ceiling Eye Roll to get the intensity down even further. Roger Callahan, the founder of TFT, used this technique, which involves holding or tapping on the same gamut point discussed above.

While tapping or gently pressing on the gamut point, keep your head level and lower your gaze to look down to where the floor meets the wall across from you, or as far down as you can look without moving your head. Slowly roll your gaze up the wall until you reach the point where the wall meets the ceiling, or as high as you can look without moving your head.

Notice your intensity level after completing this technique. The first time I used it, I was surprised by how much calmer I felt. It may sound a little "woo-woo," but give it a try.

THE PERSONAL PEACE PROCEDURE

The name, Personal Peace Procedure, just sounds relaxing, right? Having personal peace is such a great goal. With EFT tapping, personal peace is available to you with commitment and practice.

Gary Craig created the Personal Peace Procedure to help us clear out years and years of small—and not so small—negative issues that have built up. Maybe we couldn't deal with them at the time, so they're all still bottled up or hidden. Together, all these issues are collecting dust and creating a disturbance in our body's energy system. Now that you have EFT, it's time for some cleaning and clearing.[4]

To start your personal peace journey, set aside time with your tapping journal. I like to use a special journal or notebook dedicated to this Personal Peace Procedure, but it can be a separate section of an existing journal.

Start a list of all the annoying or bothersome events from the past. Each specific event counts, and because each contributes to current issues in different ways, you'll want to address them systematically; this may sound daunting but stick with me here.

Your list might have fifty, one hundred, even two hundred events. That's okay. Just think, even if you tap on one event each day, you'll have cleared many items on your list within a few months. Won't it be exciting to be free from the negative emotions associated with annoying reminders from the past?

This list won't be created, nor cleared, in a day. You can add to it anytime something else comes to mind. And as you tap, that'll definitely happen.

Start with listing childhood events. Remember that each event needs to be rather short and specific. If it's too big or too general, you might miss clearing all the subtle details and aspects. Keep them short, maybe a one- to three-minute episode that has at least one emotional peak, a beginning, an end, and specific characters. Give each event a name, such as: that time when I was six and my mom said I couldn't have a peppermint.

As you list each event, put a number next to it from 0 to 10 to indicate the intensity of emotion around the corresponding event at the time you list it. You may want to prioritize and tackle some of the mild or medium intensity events first, or maybe tap on one relatively intense event and one less intense event at a time. It might be a good idea to set a goal of tapping each day on a specific number of events, even if it's only one. Follow your instincts to find a method that works best for you.

After clearing some highly charged events, or maybe after clearing a certain number of events, mark them off your list and update the intensities of the remaining items. Thanks to the Generalization Effect[5] in EFT, as you tap through and resolve issues, other issues become less intense without having to tap specifically for them. This is yet another thing to love about EFT tapping.

Even though progress can be made quickly, continue adding to and clearing events on your list as a regular habit. It can be tempting to stop when you start feeling a little better, but please keep going. It is SO worth it!

As you clear out your old energy disruptions, you'll begin noticing subtle (and sometimes not so subtle) positive changes in your life. You may start sleeping better, eating better, feeling more confident, noticing less stress, and experiencing less frustration at home and work. You may even be smiling and feeling thankful more often. EFT can help us in countless ways if we do the easy work of tapping every single day.

That was a bunch of information, so here's a quick summary to get you started on your Personal Peace Procedure:

1. Start a list of specific bothersome events from your past.
2. Rank the intensity of each event from 0 to 10.
3. Tap on one or more events each day.
4. Review the list of events and their intensities periodically as you progress.
5. Watch for positive changes in your life!

MANAGING PAIN WITH TAPPING

"EFT is at the forefront of the new healing movement." –
Candace Pert

You've learned the basics of EFT and some additional techniques for addressing stubborn issues. And by now you understand that, if left unchecked for long enough, chronic stress will result in some sort of physical pain or illness. Let's look at a couple of the most common physical manifestations of stress: migraines and back pain.

Of course, any frequently recurring or extreme pain should be checked out with a medical professional first. **EFT tapping is in no way a substitute for professional medical advice but can be used effectively as a complementary modality**.

TAPPING FOR MIGRAINES

Migraine headaches are always painful and sometimes downright debilitating. Many migraine sufferers spend several days unable to work or even stay in an upright position. Migraines can return often, effectively stealing your precious time and robbing you of happiness. Sometimes the cause is physical, such as when we become dehydrated. Often, the cause is an emotional blockage or past trauma.

Since EFT is an evidence-based treatment that helps with physical pain and with emotional blockages, tapping can help relieve and even eliminate migraine headaches. My personal experience with using EFT for my migraines has proven it works quite well.

One of the times that EFT helped with my migraines was at the end of a stressful week away from home. I had been eating unfamiliar foods, exposed to constant exhaust fumes, as well as physically and emotionally challenging situations. The day I was to leave, I started seeing the familiar pre-migraine visual pattern. I'm one of the 25 percent of migraine sufferers who experiences a visual aura as a warning sign before the pain of a migraine begins.

This migraine was not my first; I'd been living with them for many years. But thankfully, I learned to use EFT tapping. I had used tapping to stop a migraine in its tracks before, so I decided to do that again, wondering if the first time had been a fluke.

I went into a quiet room by myself, settled down, and started tapping on the side of my hand, using *setup statements* like:

"Even though I have a migraine that's trying to start, I completely accept myself anyway."

"Even though I know my body is just trying to keep me safe by making me slow down, I accept and forgive myself."

"Even though my body is reacting to all this stress by giving me a migraine, I accept how I feel and thank my body for trying to take care of me."

Tapping on the other points, I used *reminder phrases* like:

TOH: "Thank you, body."
EB: "I know you're trying to protect me."
SE: "I've been going nonstop for seven days in a row."
UE: "And I know that's too much for me."
UN: "I hear you loud and clear,"
Ch: "and I see the aura that means a migraine is coming."
CB: "I accept that this is simply your way to help me slow down and take care of myself."
UA: "And I promise I will do that starting right now."
TOH: "I can let go of most of this stress today."
EB: "And I will plan a day of self-care and put it on my calendar."
SE: "Taking care of myself will help me be my best self."
UE: "Thank you for helping me see that I need to slow down."
UN: "I'm ready to start listening now."

Ch: "I appreciate you taking care of me."
CB: "I'm releasing this stress now so I can get through today."
UA: "Releasing all this stress now."

For this migraine, in addition to the basic recipe, I tapped on all the finger points and even threw in the 9 Gamut Procedure described in the "Additional Tapping Techniques" chapter. I tapped for about ten minutes straight, round after round, listening to and acknowledging what my body had to say. Then I was completely still for another minute. I listened to my body, breathing slowly and evenly, and started to feel calmer.

When I left the room, I made sure to drink plenty of water and started planning my day of self-care right then. My migraine never bloomed. The aura stopped and the pain never came! Even though I had used EFT tapping to stop a migraine before, it still amazed me that it really worked. And if it worked for me, it could work for you, too.

Since a migraine will most likely take you out of commission for hours if not days, ten to fifteen minutes of quiet time to tap is well worth the effort. Start early for the best results.

Thankfully, that's one of the last times I've had a migraine present itself. Maybe I've got them under control because I'm much better now at taking time out for myself and regularly practicing self-care. I recommend daily tapping, even when you don't have words. The simple act of regular tapping on the points will calm and relax you so that life becomes more balanced and manageable.

If you suffer from migraines, you can address the physical pain using the following generic *setup statement* and *reminder phrases*. As always, substitute your own specific wording that applies to the sensations of your headache and your emotions at the time.

Before you start tapping, estimate the intensity level of your headache on a scale of 0 to 10, with 0 being no pain, and 10 being the worst you can imagine. Write the number down for later comparison.

Repeat your *setup statements* while tapping on the *side of the hand* point:

> "Even though I have this migraine headache, I accept and forgive myself."

> "Even though my head is splitting and I feel terrible, I completely accept and forgive myself."

> "Even though my migraine is so painful, I love, accept, and forgive myself."

Then move through the other tapping points with *reminder phrases* such as:

> *TOH*: "This painful headache."
> *EB*: "This migraine."
> *SE*: "This nausea and headache."
> *UE*: "This awful headache."
> *UN*: "It feels like a tight band around my head."
> *Ch*: "I feel terrible."
> *CB*: "I'm so tired of this headache."
> *UA*: "This painful migraine."

After one or more rounds of tapping, take a comfortably deep breath or two and estimate the new intensity level of your pain. Write that down next to your original number. Maybe the number has decreased significantly, but if not, continue tapping to reduce the intensity level even more. If the number is not going down after repeated rounds, make sure you are well hydrated and that your words are specific to what you're feeling.

You can always try tapping on the finger points and using the 9 Gamut Procedure, as mentioned above. Ask your body what it needs or what the pain is trying to tell you. It might be time to consider that, maybe, it's not just a physical pain. It might be time to look at possible emotional causes.

If you have an idea of what brought on your migraine, such as a stressful work situation, a recent family argument, or some other traumatic event, tap specifically on that situation.

> "Even though work is really stressful for me right now, I completely accept myself."

But what if you don't have a single clue which emotions might be behind this thumper of a headache? Easy enough:

> "Even though I don't know why I have this migraine, I accept and forgive myself."

EFT is wonderful like that. By tapping on the "I don't know" statements, we can very often experience memories or insights that lead us directly to the source of our emotional disturbance. And then we tap on that.

Like the layers of an onion, we slowly peel away feelings and sensations until we've discovered the core issue(s) that can be neutralized one at a time using EFT. There is a long list of links to migraine relief success stories on the EFT Universe website.[1]

TAPPING FOR BACK PAIN

Almost everyone I know has complained of back pain at some point. It may be short-term acute pain from a sudden injury or chronic pain that lasts much longer than expected. While all physical pain is real regardless of the duration and should be evaluated by a medical professional, chronic pain often holds secrets that EFT tapping can help break through, allowing you to experience some amount of physical relief.

Yes, I have a personal story about back pain too. And much of what I reported in the migraine section applies for back pain as well. It took me too many years to figure out that much of my back pain was due to chronic stress. Years of needless suffering and limiting activities could have been avoided had I learned about EFT earlier. But once I learned how to use it effectively, I was able to say goodbye to chronic back pain and set boundaries to avoid the stress that was causing it.

If you suffer from back pain, you can approach the physical sensations directly with tapping by using the basic recipe. To find your specific words, think about the pain you're feeling and exactly where it's located. Is it in your upper, middle, or lower back? Is it on one side or both? Is it sharp or dull? Throbbing or stabbing? Does it have a color? Does it make any sound? How big is it? Is it rough or smooth? Does it have a name? (I know that seems like a strange question but try asking. You might be surprised what comes up.) Is there anything else about this pain that you can describe?

Then estimate the intensity of the pain on a scale of 0 to 10. Start tapping on the *side of the hand* point with your specific *setup statements*, followed by short, detailed *reminder phrases*. After tapping, estimate your new intensity level and write it down next to your starting number.

Continue tapping more rounds with your specific words. Incorporate any of the additional tapping techniques you've learned until you've relieved the pain as much as possible. Then ask yourself: "What's stopping this from being a 0?" Notice what comes up and tap on that. As a species, we're an intricate puzzle of emotions and feelings. EFT can help us solve the puzzle more easily.

If you're having trouble finding details to describe your back pain, start general and see what emerges. A good starting place is to estimate your intensity level and write the number down, then start tapping on the *side of the hand* point:

> "Even though I have this pain in my back, I accept myself and how I feel."

> "Even though this back pain is very uncomfortable, I love and accept myself anyway."

"Even though I'm really tired of this back pain, I am open to finding a way to release it now."

Tap through the rest of the points:

TOH: "This back pain."
EB: "I don't think it will ever go away."
SE: "And I'm so tired of it."
UE: "I wonder if it will ever stop."
UN: "I wonder why it started."
Ch: "This back pain."
CB: "Maybe it has something to tell me."
UA: "I'm ready to get to the bottom of this back pain."

Take a slow, calming breath and check in with your intensity level again. Write it next to your starting intensity. Did it change? What came up for you? Did memories or more descriptive information about the pain come to the surface? If so, tap on the new information or any specific memories and notice if that helps the pain.

Stay hydrated as you tap. Take notes often on your intensity levels and what surfaces so that you can tap on them later. Try to tap daily, if only for five minutes. It can make all the difference in lowering your overall stress and related pain.

WHEN THE PAIN RETURNS

Again, all physical pain should be evaluated by a medical professional. And you can still use EFT as a complementary approach to pain management.

Sometimes after you've used tapping successfully for pain relief and been thrilled about how well it worked for you, you may experience a return of some amount of pain. I've been there, too. My first reaction was, "What is going on?! I thought I had gotten rid of that pain!" Instead of sliding down that slippery slope of doubt, start tapping right away at the first sign of pain that's returning.

Even before you know what to say, start tapping on the *side of the hand* point. Estimate the intensity of the pain from 0 to 10, so you have a starting point. Then keep the pain at bay by tapping through a round or two. When you tap, use *setup statements* such as:

> "Even though this pain came back and I'm scared
> I'll never get rid of it, I completely accept myself."

Or use more specific words describing precisely what you're feeling and thinking. As you tap through the points, your *reminder phrases* might sound something like:

> "This throbbing red pain in the back of my head on
> the right side."

Whatever it is, be as precise as you can.

As you tap and the energy blockages begin to release, listen carefully to what comes to mind. Think back to the very first time you remember having this pain. What was going on at that time in your life? Is there anything happening now that reminds you of that time? Any people, places, smells, colors, tastes, memories that crop up? Tap on those things that create any intensity, one at a time. If there are lots of things to tap on, take the time to make a list, so you can come back to them as needed.

As I mentioned earlier, you can ask the pain and your body what it needs right now. What is it trying to tell you? Is it time to slow down, and you can't seem to make yourself take a break? Your body will help you, or make you, slow down when you don't accept that you need to. Recognize that your body is merely trying to help you in some way. Thank your body for that. Let it know you're listening.

> "Even though this headache returned, and I think
> my body is trying to tell me something, I
> completely accept myself, and I thank my body for
> trying to protect me."

Tap several rounds on what comes up for you and then estimate the intensity of your pain again. Hopefully, it has decreased. Continue tapping until you feel like you're past the worst of it and can control the pain again. Try to lower the intensity of the pain to a 0, but at least a 3 or below.

If several events or memories have come to mind, write them down for more tapping work now or schedule a time for later. Identify what you're feeling, estimate the intensity, and tap. It's quick, it's easy, and it works.

THAT PAIN IN MY NECK

One more quick story about using metaphors to get to the bottom of your pain, no matter where it is. Did you know a person or event can actually be the pain in your neck?

One day I was back at home after running errands, working with technical support on my web server errors, and tending the fire in the woodstove. I had done no heavy lifting, no awkward turns of my head, nothing that would have created the sudden sharp pain in the left side of my neck. No warning at all! I'm sitting in front of the fire, and suddenly, I can't turn my head to the left without having a sharp pain. I've had these before, and they start small and eventually run from my neck down to under my shoulder blade. And the pain can last for days.

But this was the first time I'd had one of those pains in my neck since I started EFT tapping. Aha! I could fix this now with tapping. My neck pain had an intensity level of about 8. Ouch. Tapping on the *side of the hand* point:

> "Even though I have this sharp pain in the left side of my neck at the base of my skull, I love, accept, and forgive myself."

> "Even though this pain in my neck is sharp when I look to the left, I completely love, accept, and forgive myself. And I'm okay."

> "Even though I have this sharp pain in my neck, I accept myself and I'm okay."

Tapping through the other points:

> *TOH*: "This sharp pain in my neck."
> *EB*: "Hurts especially when I look to the left."
> *SE*: "This sharp pain in my neck."
> *UE*: "Sharp pain on the left side of my neck."

86

UN: "So tired of this sharp pain in my neck."
Ch: "Really sharp pain in my neck."
CB: "Where did this pain come from?"
UA: "This sharp pain in my neck."

I could still feel it hurting, so I tried a few more rounds, talking out loud as things came up, trying to allow myself to feel safe to let it go. But the pain was still about a 6. It was time to bring out the big guns: 9 Gamut Procedure to the rescue; this worked great and brought the pain down to a 3. As I relaxed and observed how I was feeling, I tried to think about how I could get this pain down from a 3 to a 0. What came up made me laugh out loud.

The old saying "what a pain in the neck" came to mind, and in this case, what was going on in my life showed me that bothersome events and people could literally cause me to have a pain in my neck! Using that approach with my tapping language, I tried three more rounds of tapping on my stress, frustration, and disappointment about my website and email server being down after I had announced the site to lots of people. What a pain in the neck! The tapping brought the pain down to a 0. Gone. I love EFT.

If you have a particularly stubborn issue, spend time tapping on all the points, and simply allow yourself to notice or speak whatever comes to your mind. Are there any phrases emerging that might remind you of your situation? Any appropriate metaphors? If so, try using those words in your tapping. It may be exactly what you need to release the blocked energy or pain.

❧ 8 ❧

YES, BUT ...

"Put away your skepticism, this really works. I've had great results with Tapping in my own life." – Dr. Wayne Dyer

---

EFT tapping is a wonderful tool for uncovering our "Yes, but ..." thoughts and responses. What's a "Yes, but ..."?

Have you ever wondered why no matter what you do, you can't break a salary ceiling, or can't take that next step to start writing or painting? Wondered why the weight you lose keeps coming back? Wondered why you can never find Mr. or Ms. Right?

From Gary Craig: "The events in our lives create our beliefs about the world, and those beliefs can either pose limits or open new possibilities." Gary referred to these beliefs as The Writing on Our Walls.[1]

The Writing on Our Walls represents our self-talk, which reflects everything we've learned from both well-meaning or misguided authority figures throughout our lives: parents, grandparents, siblings, teachers, peers, rock stars, actors and actresses, etc. The words may or may not be true, but we have engraved them into our brains and don't question them. These become our core beliefs about ourselves and the world around us.

Our core beliefs may have served to protect us at some point in life, but now they can limit progress, keeping us stuck. You can discover your core beliefs by listening carefully to your thoughts after you state that you can do something or are open to something. Those are your silent and often invisible "Yes, but ..." thoughts.

You might say or think, "I'm going to apply for that great job! It's perfect for me." And then the Writing on Your Walls quietly reminds you, "Oh, I'm sure there are others who are more qualified. I'd never get it anyway." And then what happens? You may not even bother to apply for it, which then reinforces the Writing on Your Walls that says, "You'll never get a good job."

We've all repeated our fictional list of limits silently or aloud so many times we don't even realize we're doing it. They are our truths. So, learning to listen for our "Yes, but ..." thoughts is a significant first step in letting them go.

EFT tapping can help us erase and replace the Writing on Our Walls with more positive, hopeful, and encouraging words. Tapping helps us realize, "That was then, this is now." Tapping can help us uncover and neutralize those old limiting words and beliefs so we can move forward with our goals.

Sometimes in the tapping process, we uncover an emotionally charged event that may have put those words on our walls. If at any point you feel an issue or event is too big for you to continue working on alone, Sneak Away from the memory or emotion by tapping and saying that even though you feel this strong emotion, you'll come back to it soon with help. (There's more on Sneaking Away in the "Additional Tapping Techniques" chapter.) Consult with a certified EFT practitioner or other professional before moving forward on a traumatic event or issue so that you can safely neutralize the negative emotions and unblock the stuck energy.

You are an amazing person with unlimited potential. Allow me to say that again: you are an amazing person with unlimited potential. What "Yes, but ..." thoughts just came up for you? There's your next tapping topic!

❧ 9 ❧

INCORPORATING TAPPING
INTO LIFE

"EFT is a simple, powerful process that can profoundly influence gene activity, health and behavior." – Bruce Lipton, PhD

Initially, I learned and practiced tapping as its own thing. I practiced my breathing and meditation, I did some tapping during the day, I wrote in my gratitude journal before sleep, and I lived my life. With time and practice, however, I've learned that most of these tools work together quite well, like the old saying, "The whole is greater than the sum of the parts." I've also learned that I can incorporate them into the "live my life" portion of my days. I've always been a multitasker, so this efficient use of time makes me very happy.

Some of your other stress-relief activities may allow space to add a variation of tapping for added stress relief. For example:

- If you have a breathing practice or plan to start one, add the Breathe and Tap Technique or the Hold and Breathe Technique (both found in the "Additional Tapping Techniques" chapter) to boost the calming effect of both breathing and tapping. At first, it might be distracting, but with only a little practice, it will feel more natural and you'll notice the added benefits.
- If you have a meditation practice, while sitting in silence or during a walking meditation, you could easily add in the Hold and Breathe Technique on the finger points.
- If you have a gratitude practice of writing down several things you're grateful for each day, you might enjoy tapping on the points while re-reading your journal at the other end of the day. For example, if you write before bed, then first thing in the morning, start gently tapping while reading your previous entries, either silently or aloud. And vice versa, read your morning "gratefuls" while gently tapping before going sleep at night.

A fun way to incorporate EFT tapping into your life is to start noticing where you might be able to add tapping throughout your day. You can tap before a meeting at work, before and during a test, before an interview, when you receive bad news, are feeling sad, can't sleep, get a headache, feel the first signs of stress creeping up, are at a stoplight, or while waiting in line. When and where else can you think of using tapping?

If you're not in a place where you can comfortably use the basic recipe, such as if people can see you tapping on your head, etc., then you can find a restroom or a quiet space to tap. Or you can tap on or hold the finger points while saying the words to yourself in your mind; this is an excellent supplement to the basic recipe and certainly better than no tapping at all.

Once you have tapped enough times that you're familiar with the sensation of tapping on each of the points, you may be able to imagine tapping on those points and feel the stimulation of the endpoints of the meridians while saying the statements to yourself. You'll still receive calming benefits.

So for now, just think about where you can incorporate tapping into your life. How can you create a habit so that you start tapping automatically when you feel stressed? As you use this tool more and more, you'll realize how beneficial it is. My motto is:

"Tap early, tap often."

Even when you don't think you need to tap for anything, try tapping anyway. It's like getting a tune-up for your energy system, keeping everything clear.

As I wrote the title of this chapter, it made me think more about the phrase: tapping into life. There's no doubt in my mind that EFT tapping has given me back my life both physically and emotionally. I've literally tapped into the awareness that I have control over how I feel and how I react. I know now that the choice is mine, and with choice comes freedom. My sincere wish for you is that you choose to explore the ways that EFT tapping can help you feel better and enjoy life.

SCIENTIFIC EVIDENCE

"Research trials have shown the remarkable and positive effects of Tapping on PTSD, anxiety, depression and phobias, as well as chronic pain, fatigue, and its successful use in the cessation of smoking has also been established." – Dr. Peta Stapleton

Hardly a day goes by that I don't hear about a new article talking about the benefits of using EFT tapping. New books and videos are coming out about the science supporting EFT tapping. Articles about tapping are appearing in popular magazines and newspapers worldwide and are being talked about by famous talk show hosts on television.

Even when visiting relatives, I'm pleasantly surprised when they show me different articles in their magazines describing the tapping process and what it can be used for. This all makes me incredibly happy! I love using EFT, and the more people who know about tapping, the more who will benefit from this helpful tool.

One exciting addition to the knowledge base is a book released by Dr. Peta Stapleton from Bond University called *The Science Behind Tapping*.[1] I affectionately refer to Dr. Stapleton as the energizer bunny of EFT research. She has conducted a remarkable number of scientific studies on the efficacy of using EFT tapping for things like food cravings and weight issues, pain, stress, depression, trauma, and PTSD. She's even been repeating previous studies to add validity to the results. Some of her studies include functional magnetic resonance imaging (fMRI) of the brain before and after tapping, which show clear results of the difference EFT makes.

Dr. Stapleton's book includes the growing evidence on the positive effect of EFT tapping on study participants, both in the short and long term. She includes case studies and descriptions of the methodology. She's conducted meta-analyses, which are combined studies of multiple clinical trials, thereby yielding even greater statistical power and proof.

There is no longer any doubt that EFT tapping is a proven, effective technique for managing many physical, psychological, and emotional issues. The studies are many, and more are being conducted. My hope is that very soon, EFT tapping will be a common tool in every household. It's easy to learn, it works quickly, and it can make a positive difference in your life and the lives of your family and friends. EFT tapping works great with children! They don't care how it works; they just know they feel better after tapping. Imagine if we had a generation of kiddos who could self-regulate their stress. It's possible with EFT.

BUT IS EFT TAPPING EVIDENCE BASED?

In 2018, an international company's Health and Wellness Program Manager stated that her company could not endorse a "Lunch and Learn" session featuring Emotional Freedom Techniques because EFT was not evidence-based. I was quite stunned that EFT tapping wasn't considered worthy of being presented to a group of stressed-out workers when I knew it would be beneficial to them as a simple self-help tool.

Once I tapped about my initial reaction to this rejection and calmed down a bit, I began collecting more information about what the designation of "evidence-based treatment" entails. If you want to know more yourself, and perhaps be able to show the worth and value of EFT to someone else who's wondering about its value, below is a brief explanation and a few references.

What does "evidence based" mean? According to the Oregon Research Institute, "An evidence-based practice is a practice that has been rigorously evaluated in experimental evaluations—like randomized controlled trials—and shown to make a positive, statistically significant difference in important outcomes."[2]

There is no debate about EFT being helpful for many conditions. Many people, including myself, can provide examples of how EFT helps with stress, physical pain, phobias, test anxiety, cravings, etc. The list goes on and on. And we can definitely say that EFT is scientifically valid and that EFT meets the criteria to be considered evidence based. Until 2018, however, for a treatment to be officially called evidence based, it had to have been listed in the National Registry of Evidence-Based Programs and Practices (NREPP). NREPP was a searchable online database of mental health and substance abuse interventions and was part of the US government's Substance Abuse and Mental Health Services Administration (SAMHSA). Sadly, in 2018 the Assistant Secretary for Mental Health and Substance Use and SAMHSA phased out the NREPP website, which had been in existence since 1997.

EFT's precursor, Thought Field Therapy (TFT), had been listed by NREPP as an effective evidence-based treatment for trauma- and stress-related disorders and symptoms, such as Post-Traumatic Stress Disorder (PTSD), effective for improving self-regulation, and for improving personal resilience and self-concept. TFT was also listed by NREPP as a promising treatment for symptoms of depression, anxiety disorder, and for general functioning and well-being.[3]

Because EFT is based on TFT, works basically the same way, is shown to be beneficial, and was submitted to NREPP (before its untimely demise) with many supporting studies for consideration as an evidence-based treatment, the contributing EFT researchers had hoped that it would be only a matter of time and funding until it was also officially listed. When NREPP was dismantled, those efforts were lost.

To replace NREPP, SAMHSA created the Evidence-Based Practices Resource Center.[4] When asked in February 2020 if there was a plan to move forward with all the existing evidence that had been submitted supporting EFT as an evidence-based practice, SAMHSA provided this reply:

> *"In terms of your last question about applying to be considered evidence-based, SAMHSA's Evidence-Based Practice Resource Center (EBPRC) no longer accepts submissions from program developers or outside researchers. Instead, it now utilizes expert input from within SAMHSA and across the federal government to identify critical topics and develop salient materials. The Resource Center is part of SAMHSA's new comprehensive approach to identifying and disseminating clinically sound and scientifically based policies, practices and programs. It enables SAMHSA to more quickly develop and disseminate expert consensus on the latest prevention, treatment, and recovery science; collaborate with experts in the field to rapidly translate science into action; and provide communities and practitioners with tools to facilitate comprehensive needs assessment, match interventions to those needs, support implementation, and evaluate and incorporate continuous quality improvement processes."*

There is no mention of TFT on the current EBPRC website, using their search tools.

Meanwhile, there's a continually growing collection of publications on the effective use of EFT as a treatment for numerous conditions. "While many hybrids or variations of EFT can be found, the term Clinical EFT has emerged to refer to the EFT tapping protocols that have been validated by research, along with the knowledge base that has developed from investigations of these procedures in the treatment of various populations and conditions."[5]

Dr. Peta Stapleton stated at a conference in Spring 2018 that EFT tapping was in the top 10 percent of treatments being researched in the field of Energy Psychology. At that point, the research included more than fifty randomized controlled trials, forty pre-post outcome studies, and of those ninety-plus studies, 98 percent showed effectiveness. In addition, four meta-analyses, five systematic reviews, and hundreds of case studies contribute to the evidence that EFT works.

According to Dr. Craig Weiner on his Science of Tapping website: "Research done in 10 countries, involving 60 researchers, resulting in publication in 20 peer-reviewed medical and psychology journals have demonstrated that EFT is effective for phobias, anxiety, depression, PTSD, pain and numerous other problems."[6]

Researchers will often refer to EFT tapping as an evidence-based treatment in publications of their own findings, so confusion about the term is understandable. Their research may indeed be repeatable, randomized controlled trials showing that treatments using EFT provide statistically significant benefits over controls or similar treatments. But because EFT had not been listed in the NREPP before that program was dismantled, it was still not officially considered an evidence-based treatment in the US.

Most recently, the 2021 EFT International (EFTi) Scientific Symposium included a panel discussion with the EFTi Research Team. One of the questions discussed was, "Is EFT an evidence-based practice?"

Their conclusion is that one can say that EFT is an evidence-based practice based on the American Psychological Association (APA) definition and the fact that EFT falls under the APA umbrella as an effective Energy Psychology practice. These are words we've all been waiting to hear.

Hopefully, this helps bring a little light to the situation and the confusion surrounding the status of EFT tapping as an evidence-based practice.

Below is a small sample of the impressive articles providing evidence of EFT's effectiveness in addressing a variety of issues; this is only a small list of studies that can be used to help those who ask about the validity and the benefits of using EFT tapping. In addition, included is a list of valuable resources that have consolidated the many research articles and provide condition- and researcher-specific search options. Great work is being done, and I'm thankful to those providing additional evidence supporting the use of EFT tapping.

EFT RESEARCH HIGHLIGHTS

The effect of Emotional Freedom Techniques on nurses' stress, anxiety, and burnout levels during the COVID-19 pandemic: A randomized controlled trial[7]

Dincer B, Inangil D. The effect of Emotional Freedom Techniques on nurses' stress, anxiety, and burnout levels during the COVID-19 pandemic: A randomized controlled trial. Explore (NY). 2021 Mar-Apr;17(2):109-114. doi: 10.1016/j.explore.2020.11.012. Epub 2020 Dec 3. PMID: 33293201; PMCID: PMC7834511.

"A brief, single-session, online group intervention utilizing EFT was effective in significantly reducing stress, anxiety, and burnout."

Reexamining the effect of emotional freedom techniques on stress biochemistry: A randomized controlled trial[8]

Stapleton P., Crighton G., Sabot D., and O'Neill H.M., (2020). *Psychol Trauma*, 2020 Mar 12. doi: 10.1037/tra0000563 [Epub ahead of print]

"In a direct replication of Church, Yount, and Brooks (2012), this study examined changes in stress biochemistry and psychological distress symptoms in 53 participants randomly allocated to one of three 60-min group interventions: Emotional Freedom Techniques (EFT), psychoeducation (PE), and no treatment (NT). The Symptom Assessment-45 (SA-45) was used to assess psychological distress symptoms... The present results indicated the EFT group experienced a significant decrease in cortisol greater than the original study (-43.24%, p < .05), but these results were not mirrored by subjective reports of psychological distress. The EFT group reduction in cortisol was significantly different from that of the PE group (-19.67%), and as expected, the posttreatment cortisol level detected among the EFT group was lower than that of the NT group (2.02%)."

An Initial Investigation of Neural Changes in Overweight Adults with Food Cravings after Emotional Freedom Techniques[9]

Stapleton P., Buchan C., Mitchell I., McGrath Y., Gorton P., Carter B., 2019. *OBM Integrative and Complementary Medicine* 2019;4(1):14; doi:10.21926/obm.icm.1901010 [Epub]

> "The findings indicated EFT may decrease limbic region brain activity and reduce food related symptoms in overweight/obese individuals. This study also illuminates the neurological mechanisms at work behind the many successful outcome studies of EFT for weight loss."

Clinical EFT (Emotional Freedom Techniques) Improves Multiple Physiological Markers of Health[10]

Donna Bach, ND, Gary Groesbeck, BCIA, Peta Stapleton, PhD, Rebecca Sims, MCP, Katharina Blickheuser, PhD, and Dawson Church, PhD, (2019). *J Evid Based Integr Med. v.24*

> "Emotional Freedom Techniques (EFT) is an evidence-based self-help therapeutic method and over 100 studies demonstrate its efficacy. However, information about the physiological effects of EFT is limited...Reviews and meta-analyses of EFT demonstrate that it is an evidence-based practice and that its efficacy for anxiety, depression, phobias and PTSD is well-established. The research investigating physiological improvements after EFT intervention is limited; however, this study adds to the body of literature and suggests that EFT is associated with multidimensional improvements across a spectrum of physiological systems."

Neuropsychological correlates of an energy psychology intervention on flight phobia: A MEG single-case study[11]

Franck Di Rienzo, Elodie Saruco, Dawson Church, Sébastien Daligault, Claude Delpuech, Jean-Michel Gurret, Ursula Debarnot & Aymeric Guillot (2019). https://doi.org/10.31234/osf.io/s3hce [Epub]

"In this single-case MEG pilot study, an Emotional Freedom Technique (EFT) intervention produced regulation of brain regions exhibiting treatment effects in response to conventional psychotherapy and medication. The neural correlates of the threat response were attenuated, and heightened activation of brain frontal executive regions mediating limbic responses appraisal to stressful stimuli was recorded. These pilot results are consistent with the literature indicating that EFT is an evidence-based treatment for phobias. They provide for the first time knowledge regarding the neurophysiological mechanisms underlying the treatment effects. This study pioneers the methodology required to conduct randomized controlled trials."

World-first brain scan research shows 'tapping' effective in combating food cravings[12]

https://bond.edu.au/intl/news/49213/world-first-brain-scan-research-shows-tapping-effective-combating-food-cravings (2017)

"Bond University Clinical Psychologist, Associate Professor Peta Stapleton led the research into Emotional Freedom Techniques (EFT) or 'tapping', which is used to treat a number of conditions including chronic pain, obesity, anxiety and stress."

The Effectiveness of Emotional Freedom Techniques in the Treatment of Posttraumatic Stress Disorder: A Meta-Analysis[13]

Sebastian, B., and Nelms, J. (2017). *Explore Journal,* Volume 13, Issue 1, Pages 16–25

> "The analysis of existing studies showed that a series of 4–10 EFT sessions is an efficacious treatment for PTSD with a variety of populations. The studies examined reported no adverse effects from EFT interventions and showed that it can be used both on a self-help basis and as a primary evidence-based treatment for PTSD."

Food for Thought: A randomised controlled trial of emotional freedom techniques and cognitive behavioural therapy in the treatment of food cravings[14]

Stapleton, P., Bannatyne, A. J., Urzi, K-C., Porter, B., & Sheldon, T. (2016). *Applied Psychology: Health and Well–Being*

> "...the current study supports the suggestion that psychological interventions are beneficial for food cravings and both CBT (Cognitive Behavioral Therapy) and EFT could serve as vital adjunct tools in a multidisciplinary approach to managing obesity."

Emotional Freedom Techniques for anxiety: A systematic review with meta-analysis[15]

Clond, M., (2016). *Journal of Nervous and Mental Disease,* *204*(5), 388-395. doi:10.1097/NMD.0000000000000483

"Emotional freedom technique treatment demonstrated a significant decrease in anxiety scores, even when accounting for the effect size of control treatment. However, there were too few data available comparing EFT to standard-of-care treatments such as cognitive behavioral therapy, and further research is needed to establish the relative efficacy of EFT to established protocols."

Emotional Freedom Techniques (EFT) to reduce the side effects associated with tamoxifen and aromatase inhibitor use in women with breast cancer: A service evaluation[16]

Baker, B. Hoffman, C. (2014). *European Journal of Integrative Medicine, 7*(2), 136-142

"Statistically significant improvements in Total Mood Disturbance and anxiety, depression, and fatigue occurred at both 6 and 12 weeks, respectively, compared to baseline. In addition, mean fatigue interference and global scores, numbers of hot flushes and the hot flush problem rating score decreased at 6 and/or 12 weeks. These preliminary findings suggest that EFT may be an effective self-help tool for women with breast cancer experiencing side effects from hormonal therapies."

Efficacy of Emotional Freedom Techniques (EFT) in reducing public speaking anxiety: A randomized controlled trial[17]

Jones, S. J., Thornton, J. A., & Andrews, H. B. (2011). *Energy Psychology: Theory, Research, and Treatment, 3*(1), p 33-42

"A significant reduction in PSA as measured by Subjective Units of Discomfort was demonstrated within the first 15 minutes of treatment with EFT, with further significant reductions also demonstrated at 30 and 45 minutes. EFT was found to be a quick and effective treatment for PSA."

A systematic review and meta-analysis of randomized and non-randomized trials of Emotional Freedom Techniques (EFT) for the treatment of depression[18]

Nelms, J. & Castel, D. (2016). *Explore: The Journal of Science and Healing, 13*(6), 416-426. doi:10.1016/j.explore.2016.08.001

"The results show that Clinical EFT is highly effective in reducing depressive symptoms in a variety of populations and settings. EFT was equal or superior to TAU and other active treatment controls. The post-test effect size for EFT (d =1.31) was larger than that measured in meta-analyses of antidepressant drug trials and psychotherapy studies. EFT produced large treatment effects whether delivered in group or individual format, and participants maintained their gains over time. This meta-analysis extends the existing literature through facilitation of a better understanding of the variability and clinical significance of depression improvement subsequent to EFT treatment."

COMPREHENSIVE SEARCH-BASED RESOURCES

Below are several searchable lists we can use and to which we can refer others so that we can all keep up with the new research and scientific studies as they are published.

Association for Comprehensive Energy Psychology (ACEP)[19] provides a database searchable by scientific rigor and provides pdf downloads of studies organized by specific condition, case studies, review articles, as well as a complete list of Energy Psychology studies.

EFT International[20] (formerly AAMET International) provides a page on The Science and Research Behind EFT Tapping, which is searchable by topic, author, article type, and year published.

EFT Tapping Training[21] provides EFT Tapping Research, searchable by topic, includes editor's notes provided by Dr. Craig Weiner.

EFT Universe[22] and Dr. Dawson Church provide a list organized by type of study and then condition.

National Emotional Freedom Techniques Training Institute (NeftTI)[23] Canada's premier EFT training institute's list is organized alphabetically and grouped by specific condition or issue.

GIFT FROM TERRY

Now that you have your copy of *Emotional Freedom Techniques*, you have a powerful tool to reduce stress by tapping into the body's energy system. With practice, you'll understand how to use and customize EFT tapping to minimize the negative impacts of stress.

As a gift to you for purchasing my book, I'm offering you my free eBook called *Ten Simple Habits to Help You Break Up with Stress* (https://fromstressedtocalm.com/gift). Give yourself a little time to explore these additional ways to manage stress so you can find your happy place again.

Here's to you for taking the initiative to improve the quality of your life and the lives of those around you.

All the Best,

Terry

P.S. If you enjoyed what you learned in this book, please leave an honest review on your favorite bookstore's website. Your review will help this book to be shown to more readers. I appreciate your support!

NOTES

1. IS THIS YOU?

1. American Institute of Stress: http://www.stress.org/daily-life
2. For a good scientific article about stress and hormones, see this one from the U.S. National Institutes of Health website: https://www.ncbi.nlm.nih.gov/pmc/articles/PMC3079864/

2. THE EFT BASIC RECIPE

1. See https://web.archive.org/web/20180212004936/https:/nrepp.samhsa.gov/ProgramProfile.aspx?id=60
2. Gary Craig, founder of EFT, "Gold Standard" EFT Tapping Tutorial. See https://emofree.com/eft-tutorial/eft-tapping-tutorial.html
3. https://eftinternational.org/
4. https://eftuniverse.com/
5. https://www.neftti.com/
6. Gary Craig. See https://emofree.com/eft-tutorial-en/tapping-basics-en/what-is-eft-en.html

3. DOES TAPPING REALLY WORK?

1. Visit https://emofree.com/eft-tutorial/eft-tapping-tutorial.html and use the search bar for a specific issue.
2. Visit https://www.eftuniverse.com/faqs/about-eft-tapping-and-this-site and search for a specific issue.

4. WHAT IF ...?

1. See https://www.thetappingsolution.com/blog/the-top-5-mistakes-people-make-with-eft-tapping-and-how-to-correct-them/
2. To find an EFT International certified practitioner, visit https://eftinternational.org/discover-eft-tapping/find-eft-practitioners/

3. See https://www.emofree.com/de/eft-tutorial/tapping-tools/pain-relief.html

5. MANAGING STRESS WITH EFT TAPPING

1. To locate a certified EFT Practitioner, see EFT International or EFT Universe

6. ADDITIONAL TAPPING TECHNIQUES

1. https://www.eftuniverse.com/refinements-to-eft/touch-and-breathe-tab
2. See https://www.eftuniverse.com/refinements-to-eft/sneaking-away-from-the-problem-in-eft
3. See https://www.emofree.com/de/eft-tutorial/tapping-tools/pain-relief.html
4. See https://eftinternational.org/the-personal-peace-procedure/
5. See https://www.emofree.com/nl/eft-tutorial/tapping-roots/generalization.html

7. MANAGING PAIN WITH TAPPING

1. See https://www.eftuniverse.com/pain-management/headaches

8. YES, BUT ...

1. See https://www.emofree.com/fr/eft-tutorial/tapping-deeper/writing-walls.html

10. SCIENTIFIC EVIDENCE

1. See https://petastapleton.com/the-science-behind-tapping/
2. For more information about the definition of an evidence-based practice, see http://www.ori.org/resources/what_does_it_mean_to_be_evidencebased
3. See the link to the archived NREPP web page on TFT for more information: https://web.archive.org/web/20180212004936/https:/

nrepp.samhsa.gov/ProgramProfile.aspx?id=60#hide3

4. See https://www.samhsa.gov/ebp-resource-center

5. The Science Behind Tapping: A Proven Stress Management Technique for the Mind and Body, Stapleton, P., 2019. Penguin Random House, p.29

6. See https://www.scienceoftapping.org/

7. The effect of Emotional Freedom Techniques on nurses' stress, anxiety, and burnout levels during the COVID-19 pandemic: A randomized controlled trial

    Dincer B, Inangil D. The effect of Emotional Freedom Techniques on nurses' stress, anxiety, and burnout levels during the COVID-19 pandemic: A randomized controlled trial. Explore (NY). 2021 Mar-Apr;17(2):109-114. doi: 10.1016/j.explore.2020.11.012. Epub 2020 Dec 3. PMID: 33293201; PMCID: PMC7834511.

8. Reexamining the effect of emotional freedom techniques on stress biochemistry: A randomized controlled trial Stapleton P., Crighton G., Sabot D., and O'Neill H.M., (2020). *Psychol Trauma*, 2020 Mar 12. doi: 10.1037/tra0000563 [Epub ahead of print]

9. An Initial Investigation of Neural Changes in Overweight Adults with Food Cravings after Emotional Freedom Techniques

    Stapleton P., Buchan C., Mitchell I., McGrath Y., Gorton P., Carter B., 2019. *OBM Integrative and Complementary Medicine* **2019**;4(1):14; doi:10.21926/obm.icm.1901010. [Epub]

10. Clinical EFT (Emotional Freedom Techniques) Improves Multiple Physiological Markers of Health

    Donna Bach, ND, Gary Groesbeck, BCIA, Peta Stapleton, PhD, Rebecca Sims, MCP, Katharina Blickheuser, PhD, and Dawson Church, PhD, (2019). *J Evid Based Integr Med. v.24*

11. Neuropsychological correlates of an energy psychology intervention on flight phobia: A MEG single-case study

    Franck Di Rienzo, Elodie Saruco, Dawson Church, Sébastien Daligault, Claude Delpuech, Jean-Michel Gurret, Ursula Debarnot & Aymeric Guillot (2019). https://doi.org/10.31234/osf.io/s3hce [Epub]

12. World-first brain scan research shows 'tapping' effective in combating food cravings

    https://bond.edu.au/intl/news/49213/world-first-brain-scan-research-shows-tapping-effective-combating-food-cravings (2017).

13. The Effectiveness of Emotional Freedom Techniques in the Treatment of Posttraumatic Stress Disorder: A Meta-Analysis

    Sebastian, B., and Nelms, J. (2017). *Explore Journal,* Volume 13, Issue 1, Pages 16–25

14. Food for Thought: A randomised controlled trial of emotional freedom techniques and cognitive behavioural therapy in the treatment of food cravings
    Stapleton, P., Bannatyne, A. J., Urzi, K-C., Porter, B., & Sheldon, T. (2016). *Applied Psychology: Health and Well–Being*

15. Emotional Freedom Techniques for anxiety: A systematic review with meta-analysis
    Clond, M., (2016). *Journal of Nervous and Mental Disease, 204*(5), 388-395. doi:10.1097/NMD.0000000000000483

16. Emotional Freedom Techniques (EFT) to reduce the side effects associated with tamoxifen and aromatase inhibitor use in women with breast cancer: A service evaluation
    Baker, B. Hoffman, C. (2014). *European Journal of Integrative Medicine, 7*(2), 136-142

17. Efficacy of Emotional Freedom Techniques (EFT) in reducing public speaking anxiety: A randomized controlled trial
    Jones, S. J., Thornton, J. A., & Andrews, H. B. (2011). *Energy Psychology: Theory, Research, and Treatment, 3*(1), p 33-42

18. A systematic review and meta-analysis of randomized and non-randomized trials of Emotional Freedom Techniques (EFT) for the treatment of depression
    Nelms, J. & Castel, D. (2016). *Explore: The Journal of Science and Healing, 13*(6), 416-426. doi:10.1016/j.explore.2016.08.001

19. Association for Comprehensive Energy Psychology (ACEP): http://energypsych.site-ym.com/?Research_Landing

20. EFT International https://eftinternational.org/discover-eft-tapping/eft-science-research/

21. EFT Tapping Training http://www.efttappingtraining.com/eft-research/

22. EFT Universe https://www.eftuniverse.com/research-studies/eft-research

23. National Emotional Freedom Techniques Training Institute (NeftTI) https://www.neftti.com/about-eft-2/articles-and-research-on-eft/

ACKNOWLEDGMENTS

SPECIAL THANKS TO MY VILLAGE:

Thank you, Deb Maluk, for providing the gift of your amazing photographs as covers for this book as well as for the entire *Art of Managing Stress* series. I'm so happy to have your beautiful works on these books. Just looking at them invites calm.

Thank you, Dawn Husted, for your excellent editing and communication skills. I appreciate the ease of working with you.

Thank you again, Diana Needham and Nathan for creating beautiful covers and clear instructional images inside the book.

Thank you, Family and Friends. I appreciate your encouragement and support.

ABOUT THE AUTHOR

Terry Maluk is a stress-management coach and author of multiple bestselling books that provide methods for learning to reduce stress and rediscover joy. A member of the American Holistic Nurses Association, Terry holds a Master of Science degree in Public Health, is an accredited, certified Emotional Freedom Techniques (EFT Tapping) practitioner, and a registered yoga teacher. Her extensive experience and her passion for helping others make her books excellent resources for anyone ready to start their journey toward a happier life.

FromStressedToCalm.com

ALSO BY TERRY MALUK

Rx for RNs: A Step-by-Step Guide to Manage Stress, Reduce Overwhelm, and Conquer Burnout

33 Nurses: Insight, Inspiration, and Stories from the Field

∾

The Art of Managing Stress Series:

Take One Breath: The Art of Managing Stress Through Mindful Breathing

In This Moment: The Art of Managing Stress Through Meditation

Emotional Freedom Techniques: The Art of Managing Stress Through EFT Tapping

Made in the USA
Coppell, TX
12 April 2023

15541461R00075